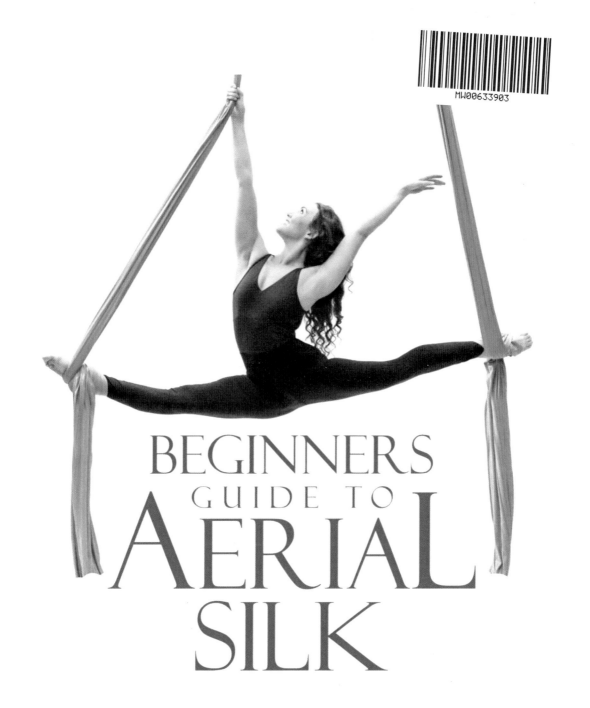

BEGINNERS
GUIDE TO
AERIAL
SILK

—— JILL FRANKLIN ——

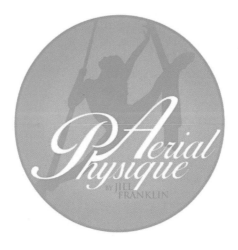

Beginners Guide to Aerial Silk
Copyright © 2017 Aerial Physique Inc.

Printed in the United States of America
ISBN: 978-0-692-28823-8

Please Note:
This book has been written and published strictly for informational purposes, and in no way should it be used as a substitute for live instruction with a professional.

TABLE OF CONTENTS

USE THIS BOOK AT YOUR OWN RISK

Aerial work is a dangerous activity that can lead to serious injury or death. The use of this book and contents therein, is at your own risk. *Beginners Guide to Aerial Silk* by Jill Franklin is intended for use as a tool of reference for those who are taking aerial classes with a live professional instructor. Always practice on aerial apparatus installed by a professional rigger, rigged from an overhead anchor graded to hold an absolute minimum of 5,000 pounds. Be sure to place a thick crash mat underneath you during practice. DO NOT practice without the supervision of a trained professional.

PREFACE

Dear Aspiring Aerialist,

My romance with aerial began many years ago when I saw my first Cirque du Soleil show at the age of fourteen. I was mesmerized by the beauty, grace and strength the performers displayed. At the time I assumed one would have to grow up in a circus school, spending hours a day training away to achieve such skill. I only had a background in ballet and did not possess the skill set to duplicate what I had admired on stage. Little did I know then, that years later I would be performing similar aerial feats in front of thousands of people in beautiful theaters throughout the world.

When I first began aerial in my early 20s in New York City, I was terrible. I lacked the upper body strength and coordination. With consistent practice, patience and belief in myself, I eventually overcame my limits with strength and achieved my skill on a professional level.

I have a passion for helping others and feel the same romance that I do with aerial. My background in ballet, classical Pilates and yoga all encompass my Aerial Physique technique. The key to any worthwhile fitness endeavor is strength, flexibility and cardiovascular activity. Aerial work has it all! The best part about it, it's incredibly rewarding and fun!

The book I have designed is for the beginner who would like to deepen their understanding of aerial silk work. It is not intended as the sole learning avenue. It is best to always practice with a qualified instructor. I wish for you to be patient, consistent and kind to yourself while learning. Enjoy, be safe and most of all have fun!

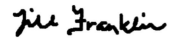

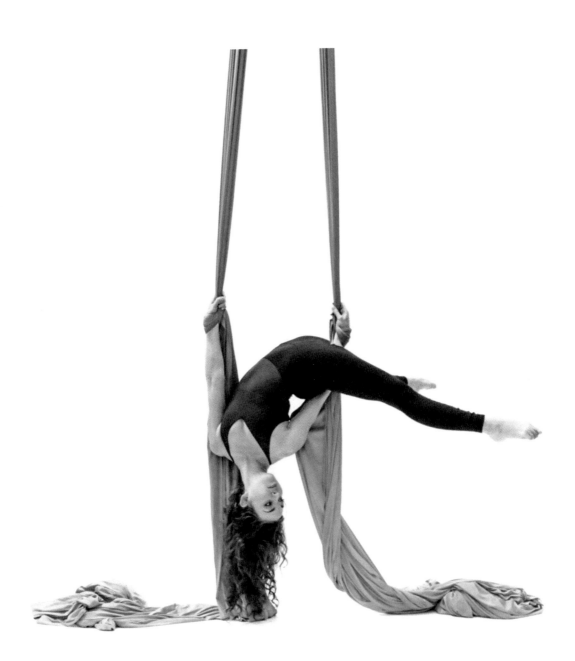

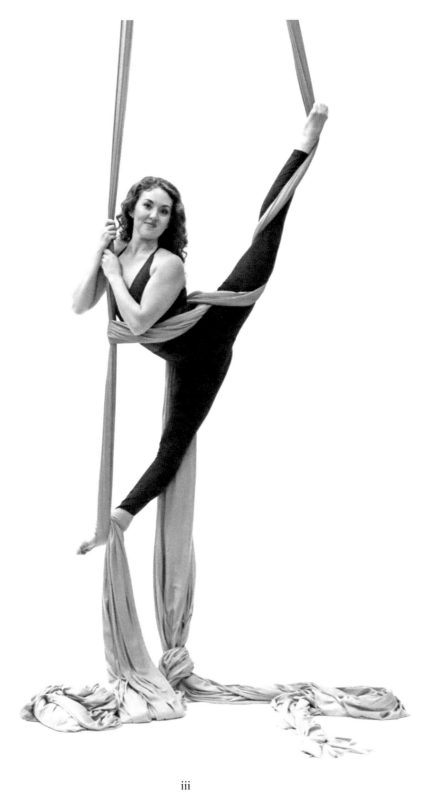

INTRODUCTION

What is aerial silk? Aerial silk (aka: fabric, tissu, ribbons) is a beautiful art form and evolving fitness craze. Practitioners of this strength building craft climb, invert and wrap their bodies into and out of various positions stemming from gymnastics and ballet. It can also be referred to as aerial acrobatics, aerial dance or aerial fitness.

Aerial acrobatics has been seen in the circus for thousands of years. The modern world began to take note of this stunning art form in 1998 when Cirque du Soleil's show *Quidam* displayed an aerial silk contortion act on red fabric. Since then, many circus schools, dance companies and most recently fitness studios and gyms have been offering classes in aerial silk.

This book introduces you to the fundamental skills, positions and movements involved in aerial silk work. The aerial movement principles are inspired by the Pilates Method principles. It also gives you an at home guide to strengthen your upper body and core when not at aerial class. The positions and movements demonstrated in this book are shown on the right side, it is important to do them on the left also. I have come across many different names for the movements and positions in this book, you may have learned them as another name. Feel free to call them what you'd like, aerial is constantly evolving.

The ascent into artistry demonstrated within, are building blocks for more advanced variations and combinations. Take your time learning the basics thoroughly, with clean technique and proper form. It is much more impressive to do the feats smooth and controlled, versus throwing yourself into things too soon and potentially getting injured or tangled in the fabric!

Keep an eye out for more Aerial Physique books and products. Visit www.aerialphysique.tv for instructional videos with Jill Franklin. For more information visit the Aerial Physique website at www.aerialphysique.com.

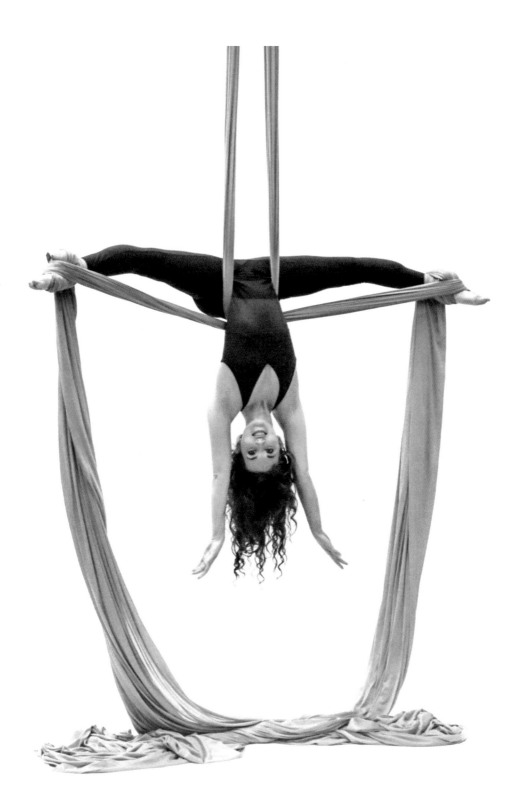

AERIAL FOUNDATION

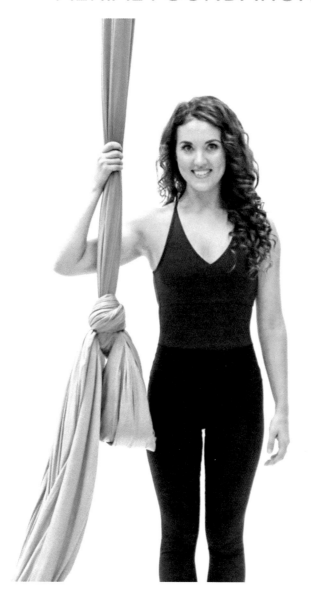

Aerial Movement Principles

1. Safety: Aerial is a potentially dangerous activity that can cause injury or even death. Make sure that you are suspended on an apparatus that has been installed by a licensed rigger and always practice with a professional instructor. Know you limits. If you find you are tired stop and rest. It is best to be safe then push yourself too far.

2. Concentration: The key element to connecting your mind and body is concentration. Aerial work is both a physical and mental practice. It is extremely important to be present in your mind while learning and executing movements. You will progress much more rapidly while having a safer approach to the task at hand.

3. Precision: Proper form is essential to ensure you achieve the beautiful lines of the positions while preventing injury.

4. Control: In aerial work, control of your entire body is the name of the game. No sloppy or haphazard movements are allowed.

5. Centering: By paying attention to the muscles of the core (abdominals, lower back, hips and glutes) you will help all of your bodies' muscles function and develop more efficiently.

6. Breathing: Controlling your breath with deep exhalations as you perform aerial movements helps activate your muscles and keep you focused. When you are upside down it is very easy to forget to breath!

7. Balance: A truly balanced body has an equal amount of strength and flexibility. Muscles should be supple, mobile, yet strong. Flexibility and range of motion are important components in aerial work.

8. Flow: In time, aerial work becomes continuous flowing movement; an *aerial dance*. Each movement, position and transition should be smooth and graceful. In the beginning movements may feel awkward and jerky, allow yourself plenty of practice and soon you will be flowing with ease!

Aerial Terminology

Aerial: Performed in the air.

Arabesque: A ballet position made by balancing on the supporting leg, while extending the free leg behind with a straight knee.

Attitude: A ballet position made by standing on one leg, while the other leg is lifted and turned out with the knee bent at approximately a 90 degree angle.

Carabiner: A metal loop with a spring-loaded gate used in rigging aerial apparatus.

Crochet: A term used in aerial silk work when wrapping your arms or legs from the outside around the fabric and securing the position using your hand or foot.

Foot Positions: The positioning of the feet is particularly important in aerial. Your feet will be pointed in most cases to finish the line of the positions. For some positions flexed or sickled feet will be an anchor in which you are hanging from.

Pointed Foot   **Flexed Foot**   **Sickled Foot**

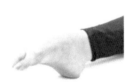 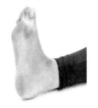 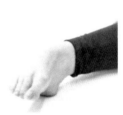

Passé: A classical ballet term meaning "passed." It refers to the movement when a dancer goes through a retiré position, which is when one leg is bent so it looks like a triangle with the foot placed near the other leg's knee.

Pike: A gymnastics term meaning bent forward at the hips.

Pilates: A physical fitness system developed in the early 20th century by Joseph Pilates. He called his method "Contrology" the art of control.

Pole of the silk: The secure or tight part of the fabric. Usually referring to the piece of fabric above your locked point (foot lock, hip key, ect.). AKA: Live End

Rescue 8: An aerial hardware piece which the fabric is wrapped around.

Rond de Jambe: A French ballet term meaning circular movement of the leg.

Rosin: A form of resin derived from pine trees, used to help gripping ability in aerial work. It is available in powered and spray forms.

Silks: A term for the fabric used in aerial work. The fabric type is commonly a strong two way stretch nylon tricot. It comes in an array of colors and stretch depending on the needs of the aerialist.

Splits: A position in which the legs are in line with each other and extended in opposite directions.

Straddle: A position in which the legs are open towards a V shape or wider.

Swivel: A hardware piece used in rigging single point aerial apparatus. It keeps the fabric in rotation and prevents it from getting twisted when in use.

Tail of the silk: The dangling part of the fabric that is below your locked point. AKA: Dead End

Tissu: Translates into "fabric" in French.

The following symbols will be seen throughout the book:

⭐ **Final Position**

 Incorrect

TIPS The tip box provides helpful tips & more details

AKA What the skill may also be known as

Your Aerial Muscles

Aerial work utilizes primarily the upper body and abdominals. Pictured below are some of the large muscles that are worked when doing aerial activities. Although in some movements the entire body is engaged, these are the main muscles at work.

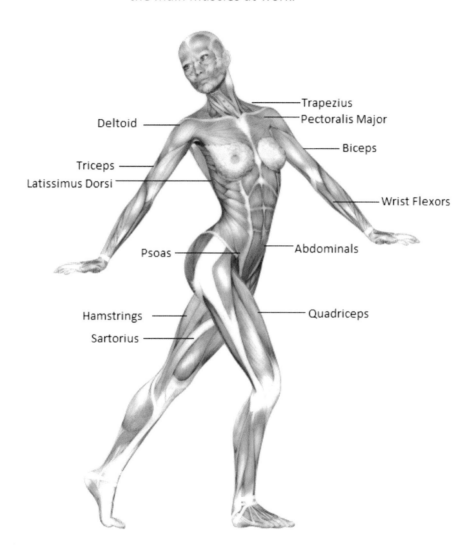

Abdominals: There are four muscles that make up the abdominal wall. All are extremely important in aerial work. **Transverse**, the deepest of the four assists in stabilizing the spine and forcing air out of the lungs. The **internal and external obliques** assist in rotating, flexing and side bending movements. Lastly the **rectus,** also known as the "six pack", works to flex (bend) the trunk.

Biceps: The front of the upper arm, it bends and supinates (turns palm upwards) the forearm. It is active during chin ups.

Deltoid: A shoulder muscle that assists in lifting the arm away from the body.

Hamstrings: A group of three muscles in the back of the leg that bend the knee and extend (straighten) the thigh. When flexible, this muscle group makes achieving a pike position is easy.

Latissimi Dorsi: Meaning "Widest Back Muscle" it is your climbing and pull up muscle. Also known as the "lats", your wings in aerial.

Pectoralis Major: Your main chest muscle, at work when doing push-ups.

Psoas: Deep hip flexor muscle that flexes the thigh and turns out the leg.

Quadriceps: The front of your thigh. A group of four muscles that assist in straightening the knee and flexing the thigh.

Sartorius: The inner thigh. It is the longest muscle in the body which works to turns out the hips. When flexible achieving a straddle position is easy.

Trapezius: Upper, middle and lower traps work to move the shoulder blades up and down. They also work when holding the arm to the side or overhead.

Triceps: The back of the upper arm, it extends (straightens) the forearm. At work in many aerial feats.

Wrist Flexors: The forearm. Bends wrists towards the body. They are your grip muscles in aerial and are worked tremendously!

PREPARING FOR AERIAL

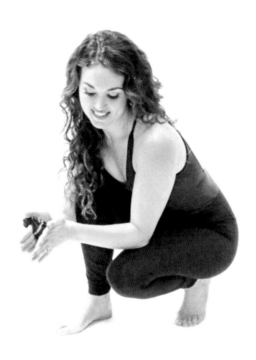

Warming Up

It is highly important to include a proper warm up prior to any aerial activities. An effective warm up heats the body and includes movements in all ranges of motion including flexion (forward bending), extension (back bending), side bending and twisting. A Pilates, ballet or gymnastics based warm up are all great options. You could also do something as simple as jogging in place or jumping jacks followed by the strength building positions and stretches as pictured in the pages to come.

Core strength is crucial in aerial work. The position below shows the correct alignment during core work or in Pilates terms your 'Powerhouse'. Proper recruitment of your abdominals, lower back, hips and glutes are all vital when working your core. A similar position is done on the fabric called the 'candlestick'. Refer to the at home guide beginning on page for more strengthening movements that are also great to incorporate in a warm up.

Core Stabilization – Hollow Body Position

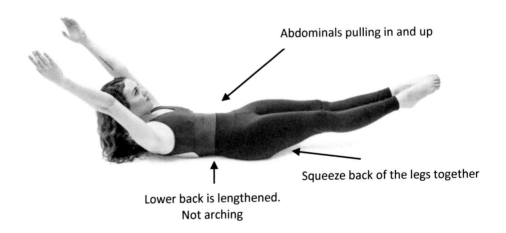

Abdominals pulling in and up

Squeeze back of the legs together

Lower back is lengthened.
Not arching

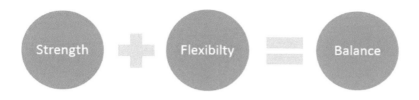

Proper Plank Position

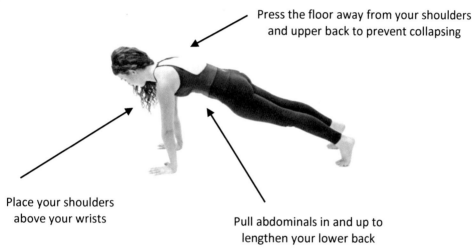

Press the floor away from your shoulders
and upper back to prevent collapsing

Place your shoulders
above your wrists

Pull abdominals in and up to
lengthen your lower back

Incorrect Plank Position

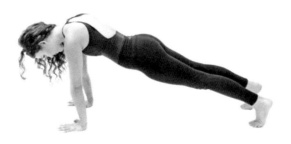

Stretching

Seated Pike

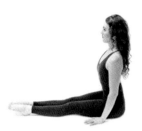 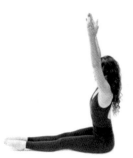 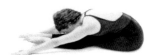

Straddle

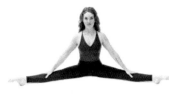 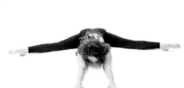 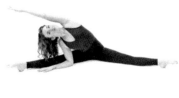

Splits

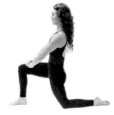 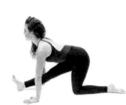 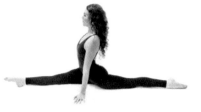

Back Bending   **Forearm Stretch**

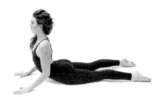 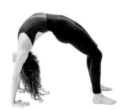

Grip & Shoulder Placement

Proper Grip

Always grip the fabric with your thumb wrapped around

Incorrect Grip

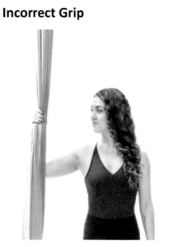

Correct Shoulder Placement

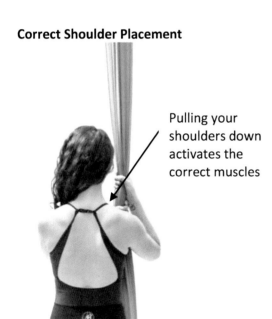

Pulling your shoulders down activates the correct muscles

Incorrect Shoulder Placement

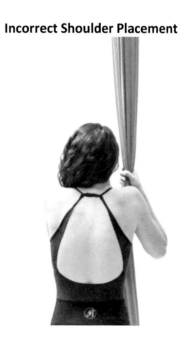

When practing aerial it is important to always remember these two fundamental components.

AERIAL SILK BASICS

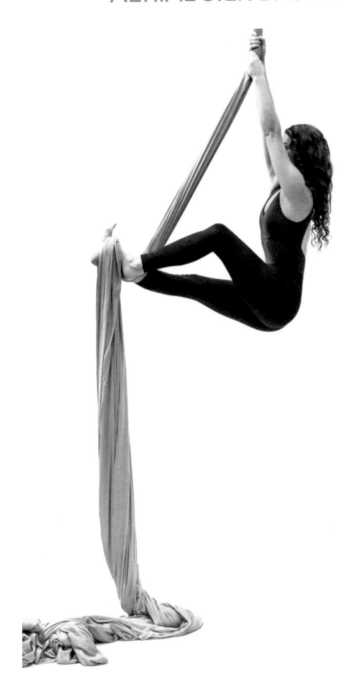

Shoulder Shrugs

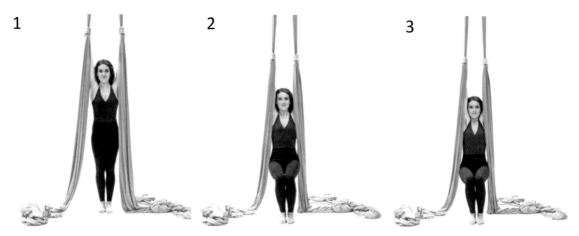

1
Begin standing between the fabrics with your arms reaching up high.

2
Step your feet approx. 1 foot forward and sit your hips back into a chair position. Pull your front ribs together and engage your core.

3
Allow your shoulders to shrug by your ears without losing the connection to your core.

Progression

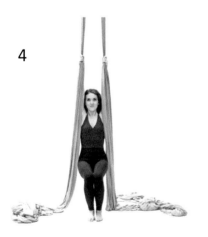

4
Draw your shoulder blades down your back. Repeat 10x.

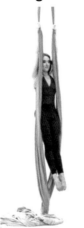

Try it in the air.

TIPS
*Shoulder shrugs are a preparatory exercise and warm-up the muscles in your upper back and shoulders for aerial work
*Proper shoulder placement when reaching arms overhead should be in between the two extremes of shrugging your shoulders and pulling them down away your ears
*As this becomes easier try the progression in the air from one climb up

Classic Climb Preparation

1

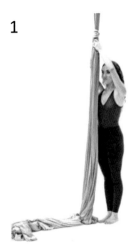

Stand next to the fabric.
Reach your arms up with
your right hand on top.

2

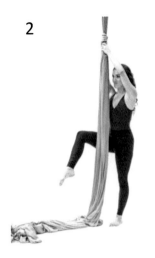

Wrap your right leg
around the fabric
from the outside in.

3

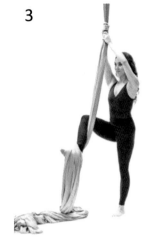

Flex your right foot creating
a step for your left
foot to stand on.

Incorrect Leg Wrap

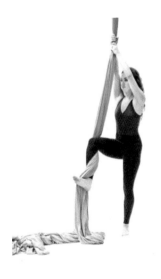

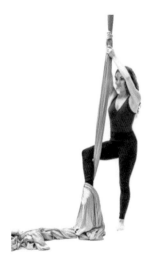

Classic Climb

1

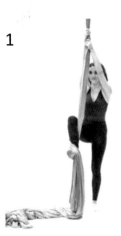

Begin in the classic climb preparation position.

2

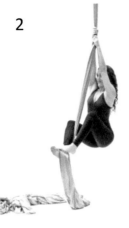

Maintaining long arms, transfer your weight into your hands while stepping the ball of your left foot on top of your right into a squat.

3

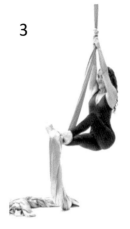

Press your feet forward and lengthen your legs creating an L shape.

4

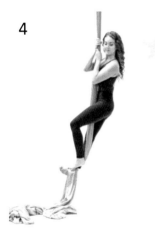

Firmly press your feet together as you pull your torso close to the fabric to an upright position.
*Steps 1-4 may be enough until you build more strength.

5

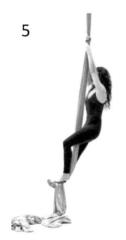

Reach your arms up high one hand a time. Tuck your hips under to engage your core.

6

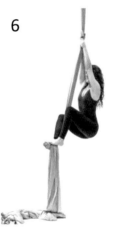

Lift your knees towards your chest while wrapping your right foot around the fabric from the outside in. Step your left foot on top of your right.

6

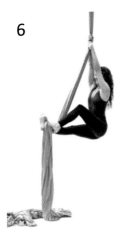

Press your feet forward and lengthen your legs creating an L shape.

7

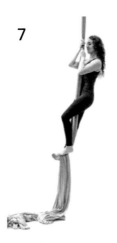

Firmly press your feet together as you pull your torso close to the fabric to an upright position.

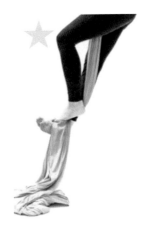

Using your legs and firmly pressing your feet together will prevent slipping and give you adequate power from your legs to help you climb.

TIPS
*Practice climbing on both sides
*Whichever leg is wrapped that is the hand that is on top
*When moving from step 1 to step 2, keep your lifted knee in line with your hip as you transfer your weight into your hands and step up
*On each climb let go of fabric with your feet and re-wrap
*The height of the climb comes from lifting your knees high toward your chest rather than pulling up with your arms
*Keep your shoulders drawing down away from your ears to ensure correct alignment and muscle recruitment
*Tucking your hips under while you lift your knees to your chest during steps 5-6 will allow your abs to initiate the movement
*This climb is a transfer of weight from your upper to lower body. Allow your legs to help you!

Advanced Challenge:
Add a pull-up between each climb versus hanging with straight arms

AKA: French Climb

Classic Climb Descent

Version #1 Squatting Decent

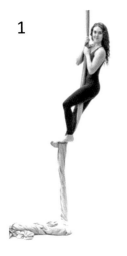

1

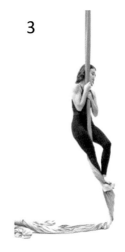

2

3

Begin from the classic climb position with your hands in front of your chest.

Sit on your heels keeping the fabric in between your legs.

Move your hands in front of your chest. Lengthen your legs and repeat.

Version #2 Hand over Hand Decent

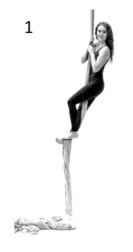

1

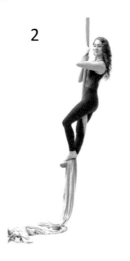

2

Walk your hands down the fabric while lightening the tension between your feet.

TIPS
*To avoid painful fabric burns be sure NOT to slide your hands down the fabric
*Never jump off of the fabric from a climbing position, instead, quietly step down once you are close to the mat
*There are several ways to descend down the fabric, these two are the most basic

Russian Climb

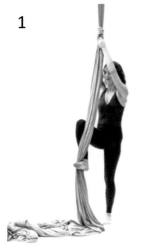

1

Place your right foot on the inside of the fabric. Firmly flex your foot.

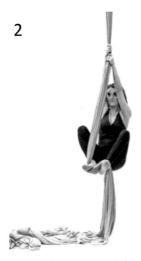

2

Transfer your weight into your hands as you scoop up the tail of the fabric with your left foot.

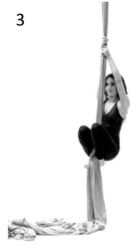

3

Step your left foot on top of your right arriving in a squat with the fabric in between your legs.

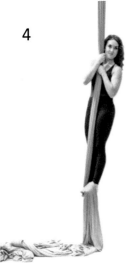

4

Press your feet together while you lengthen your legs to stand up.

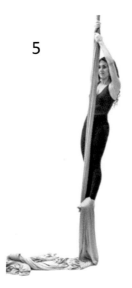

5

Reach your arms up and repeat steps 1 -4.

TIPS
*To begin, place the fabric on the outside of your lifted foot and inside your knee
*When learning this climb perform it with straight arms, as your strength improves add a pull-up
*Repeat on your other side
*To descend, re-wrap your feet in the classic climb position and use version #1 or #2 or page 17

Tying the Hammock Knot

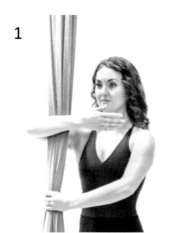

1

Hug the fabric with your right forearm.

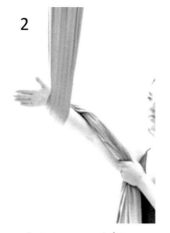

2

Rotate your right arm upwards passing your hand to the opposite side.

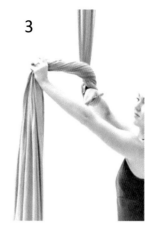

3

Loop the tail around the top fabric pulling it tightly with your left hand.

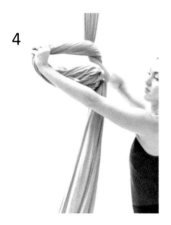

4

Keep holding the tail with your left hand. Grab the tail with your right hand to form a loop.

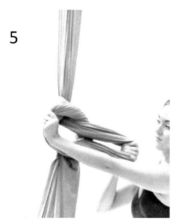

5

Grab the fabric underneath your right wrist with your left hand. Pull the loop through the hole with your right hand.

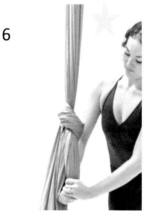

6

Pull down on the loop to make a secure hammock knot.

TIPS
*The hammock knot is used to make the two pieces of silk into a hammock
*This is a great tool to use when learning how to invert, it will help improve your coordination when upside down
AKA: Egg Knot, Slip Knot, Sling

Hammock Straddle Inversion

1

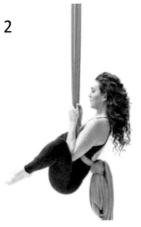

Place the hammock behind you like a backpack.

2

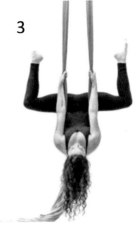

Transfer your weight into your arms. Open your legs in a frog shape, push the fabric forward while leaning your shoulders back.

3

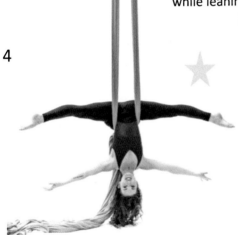

End with the hammock knot on your lower back and the inside of your thighs pressing forward against the fabric.

4

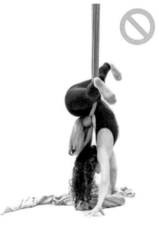

Extend your legs to the side in a straddle. Let go of the fabric and open your arms to the side.

Incorrect Position

TIPS
*Once you are inverted in the straddle position look straight ahead. Looking down not only misaligns your spine, it can make you feel dizzy and disoriented
*Press your inner thighs into the poles of the fabric to secure your straddle position
*Tuck your pelvis slightly under to avoid arching in your lower back
*To exit, retrace your path and step down lightly

1

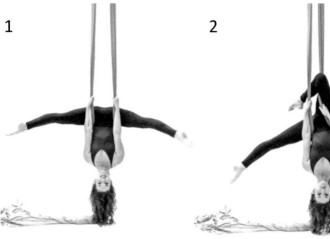

Begin from the straddle inversion position. Hold the left fabric with your left hand.

2

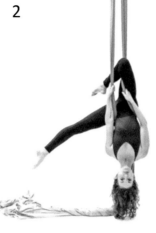

Hook the back of your right knee on the right fabric.

3

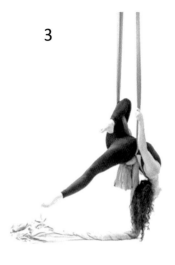

Circle your left leg behind you in an arabesque position.

4

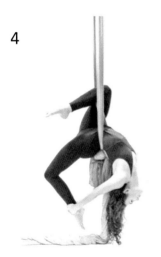

Bend your left leg and grab the front of your shin with both hands.

5

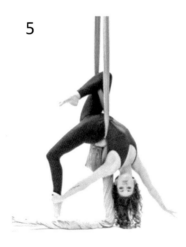

If your shoulder mobility is limited, grab your shin with one hand instead of both.

TIPS
*After the first side return to the straddle and hook your opposite knee
*Hook the back of your knee, not your foot
*Keep your hips square to the ceiling
*Once your leg has circled behind you relax your neck
*This is a great stretch for your shoulders and hip flexors!

Wrist Locks

Version #1 Straps Lock

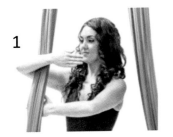

1

Hug the fabric placing it on the inside of your right wrist.

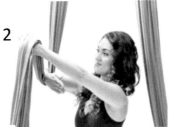

2

Using your left hand flip the fabric over your wrist.

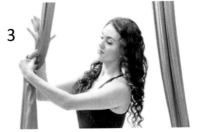

3

Turn the palm of your right hand in toward the fabric and grab.

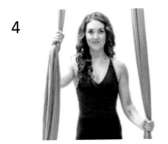

4

Grab the opposite fabric with your left hand approx. 1 foot lower than your right hand.

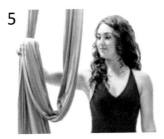

5

Join the fabrics together passing the loop to your right hand.

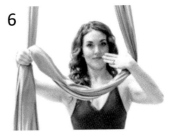

6

Place your left wrist in the loop.

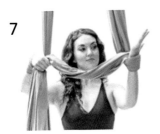

7

Circle your left wrist down around the fabric.

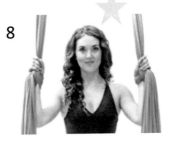

8

Pull down and grab the poles of the fabric with the tails on your pinky finger side.

Version #2 Figure 8 Lock

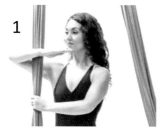

1

Hug the fabric placing it on the inside of your right wrist.

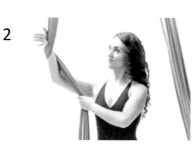

2

Begin to circle your right wrist up and around the pole.

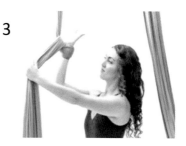

3

Using your left hand pass the tail up and over your wrist.

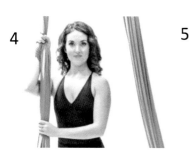

4

Pull down and grab the pole of the fabric.

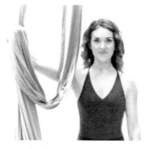

5

Grab the left fabric with your left hand approx. 1 foot lower than your right hand. Pass it to your right hand.

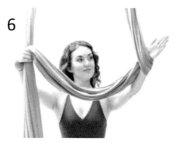

6

Place your left wrist in the loop and circle up and around.

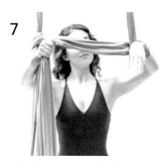

7

Using your right hand pass the tail up and over the top of your left wrist.

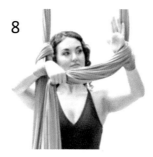

8

Circle your left hand down and around.

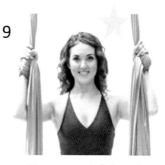

9

Turn your left hand to face the pole end and grab. The tails should face your thumb side.

Version #3 Double Wrap

1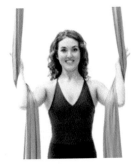

Begin standing between the
fabrics. Hug the fabric from
the outside in and circle your
wrists upward.

2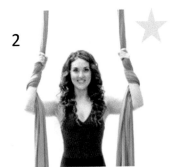

Circle your wrists one
more time to complete
two wraps.

TIPS
*The wrist locks help to support your grip strength
*The flatter you make the fabric around your wrists the more comfortable it will feel,
twisted fabric can be painful!
*As your grip strength improves you can do the movements in the pages to come
without wrist locks
*Version #1 is called Straps Lock because it is a common wrap used on aerial straps
*Version #2 Figure 8 Lock is a more secure wrap and is used when aerialists perform
flying acts on the fabric
*Version #3 Double Wrap is the least supportive of the options

"Physical fitness is the first requisite of happiness."
Joseph Pilates

Foundational Shapes

Upright Tuck

1

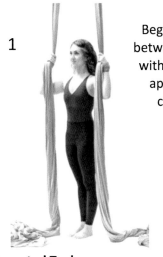

Begin standing in between the fabrics with wrist locks at approximately cheek level.

2

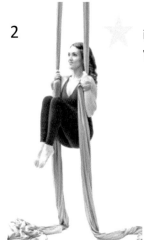

Transfer your weight into your hands, draw your elbows into your sides and lift your knees toward your chest. Hold for 3-10 seconds. Repeat 2-3 times.

Inverted Tuck

1

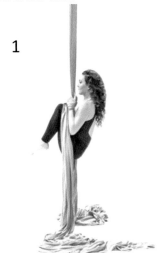

2

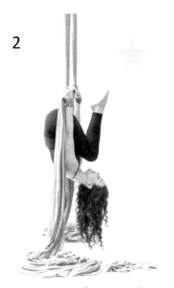

3

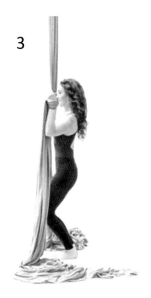

Stand between the fabrics with your wrists locked. Pull your elbows to your sides while lifting your knees to your chest. Begin to rotate backward.

Rotate until your tush is facing the ceiling. When you arrive upside down lengthen your arms.

Retrace your path to exit. Pull-up with your arms and quietly step down.

Candlestick   **Incorrect Position**

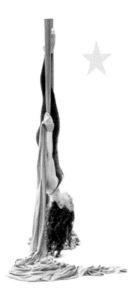   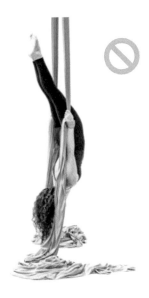

Begin from the inverted tuck. Lengthen   Be sure not to arch your back. Keep
your legs upward keeping your   your pelvis slightly tucked under,
hips and feet in between the fabrics.   abdominals in and back lengthened in
                                               hollow body position.

TIPS
*The inverted tuck can take some time to achieve due to fear of rotating
backward and lack of upper body/core strength. Continue to practice the
upright tuck until you can hold for several seconds
*Maintain a long neck, shoulder blades gliding down your back and place
elbows under your shoulders during the upright tuck and when passing
through it for the inverted tuck
*Be cautious when exiting the inverted tuck and candlestick. The floor comes
quickly! Hold your knees in a tuck and pull up with your arms to avoid a heavy
landing
*When beginning, look up at your body when you arrive in candlestick
position, looking at the floor may make you disoriented and can lead to
flipping the wrong way

AKA: Egg Roll (tuck), Pencil (candlestick)

Bird's Nest

1
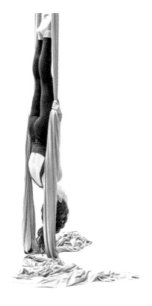

2
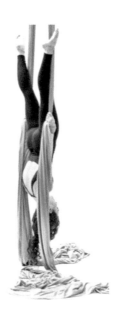

3
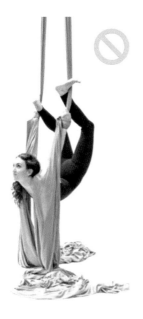

Begin in candlestick position.

Open your legs and place your shins on the back side of poles of the fabric.

Press your shins into the poles and lift your chest in the opposite direction.

Incorrect Position

TIPS
*To exit the Bird's Nest retrace your path. Pass through candlestick, tuck and lightly step down
*This is a great stretch for the front of the chest and the back
*Make sure you don't sink too low that you compress your lower spine. Instead, initiate arch from your upper back not your lower back
*This shape is used as an exit for more advanced skills such as Fallen Angel Drop

AKA: Basket, Cradle

Side Arch

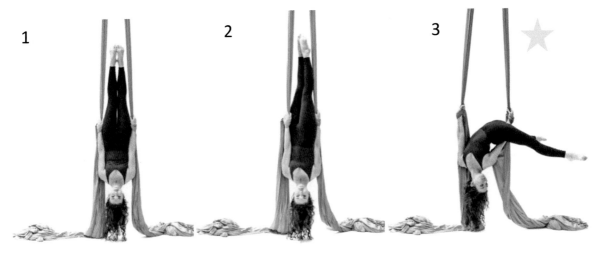

1

Begin in candlestick position.

2

Turn your hips to the side and open your legs on either side of the fabric.

3 ⭐

Lower your legs behind you until you arrive in a side arch position while keeping your hips square.

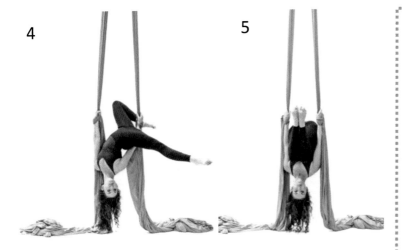

4

To exit, begin to bend your back leg toward your chest followed by your front leg.

5

End in a tuck position. Repeat on the other side.

TIPS
*A thorough back and hip flexor warm-up is important before practicing this skill
*Relax your neck once you arrive in the side arch position and look toward your legs
*It is common to get disorientated in this position, keep practicing!
*Don't forget to breathe!

AKA: Banana Boat

STRADDLE INVERSIONS

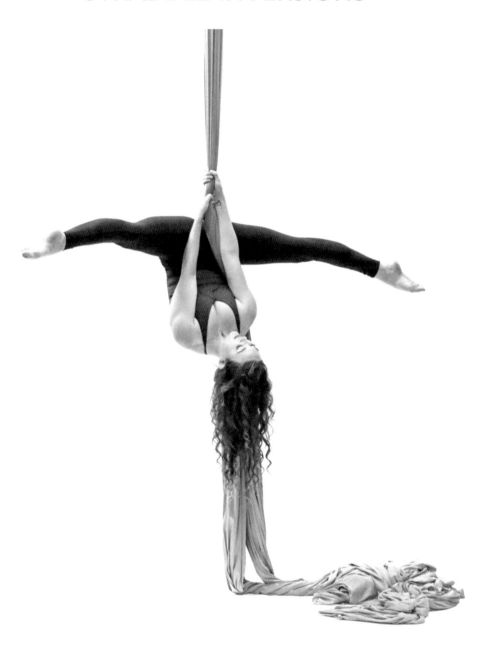

Split Fabric Straddle Inversion Prep

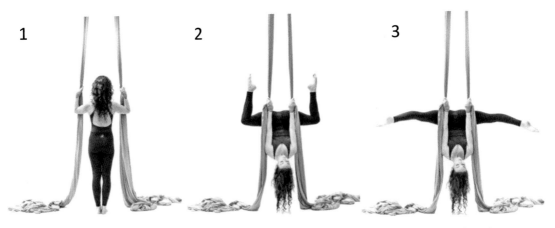

1

Begin standing between the fabrics with wrist locks on.

2

Rotate backward bending your elbows into your sides and passing through a frog shape with your legs. Arrive with your inner thighs pressing against the fabrics and your arms lengthened.

3

Unfold your legs into a straddle. Press your forearms toward your inner thighs and slightly tuck your pelvis under. Retrace your path to exit.

Correct Position

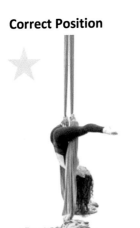

Incorrect Position

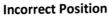
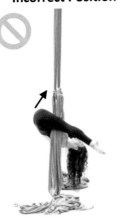

TIPS
*This is more challenging than the inverted tuck
*Lift your pelvis up toward your hands, no drooping bums allowed!
*Once you arrive in the straddle keep your focus on your hands, not on the floor, looking down misaligns your spine
*Palms and forearms should be turned to face your inner thighs
*When you feel confident with this position do it without wrist locks
*To exit, retrace your path and step down lightly

1

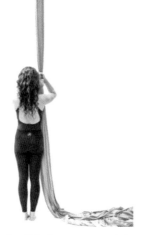

Begin with the fabric on your right with your right hand on top.

2

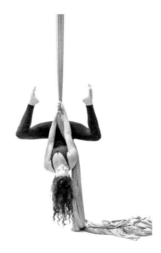

Rotate backwards bending your elbows into your sides and passing through a frog shape with your legs. Arrive with your inner thighs pressing against your forearms and your arms lengthened.

3

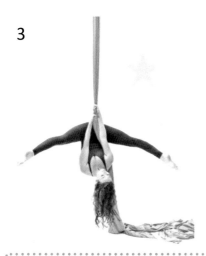

Extend your legs into a straddle.

TIPS
*This is a very important skill to achieve! Eventually this turns into inversion climbs and the beginning of many tricks
*When you become stronger passing through a frog position is not necessary, you can keep your legs straight the entire time
*Repeat on the other side with the opposite hand on top
* To exit, pull up with your arms, retrace your path and step down lightly

Invert & Hook

1

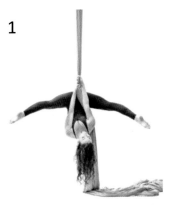

Begin in a straddle inversion with the tail to the right.

2

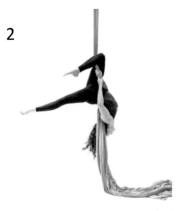

Hook the back of your right knee and rotate your left leg behind you. This is known as 'Same Side Hook'.

3

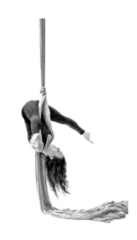

Return to a straddle.

4

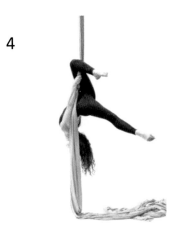

Hook the back of your left knee on the fabric and rotate your right leg behind you. This is known as 'Opposite Side Hook'.

5

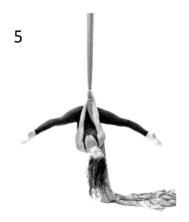

Return to a straddle.

TIPS
*Lift your pelvis up toward your hands during each straddle inversion
*Perform a slight pull up from your latissimus dorsi muscles prior to hooking your knee to avoid hooking your knee on top of your hands
*When the fabric is on your right side and you hook your right knee, that is referred to as Same Side Hook. When the fabric is on your right side and you hook your left knee, that is referred to Opposite Side Hook, vice-versa

Bent Leg Straddle Inversion

1

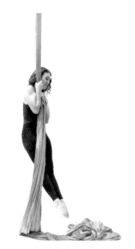

Begin from a classic climb with your hands in front of your chest, right hand on top and elbows into your sides.

2

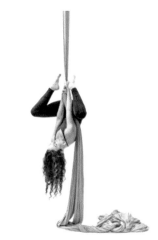

Release your feet while turning your hips away from the fabric. Keep the tail on the outside of your right hip.

3

Initiate the inversion by tucking your hips under and drawing your elbows into your sides as you rotate backwards passing your legs through a frog shape.

4

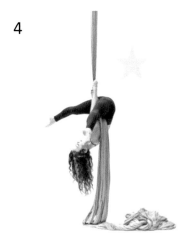

Extend your legs into a straddle.

5

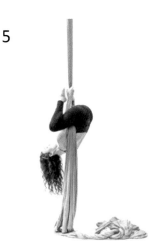

Begin retracing your path.

6

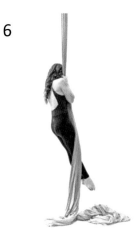

Draw your elbows toward your hips and pass through hollow body. Repeat or rewrap in classic climb.

Straight Leg Straddle Inversion

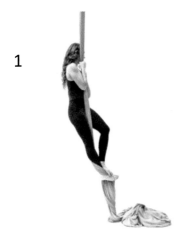

1

Begin from classic climb with your hands in front of your chest, right hand on top and elbows into your sides.

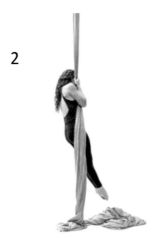

2

Release your feet while turning your hips away from the fabric. Keep the tail on the outside of your right hip.

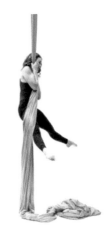

3

Initiate the inversion by tucking your hips under and drawing your elbows into your sides. Rotate backward maintaining engaged and straight legs.

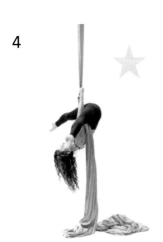

4

Extend your legs into a straddle. Retrace your path to exit. Repeat or rewrap in classic climb.

Incorrect Position

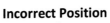

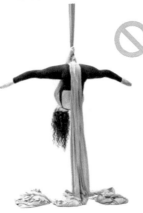

The fabric is in between the legs and not to the side.

TIPS

*Passing your legs through a frog shape will make it easier to get your hips over your head. In time, work towards inverting with straight legs

*Do your best to keep your arms bent and elbows into your sides while inverting, if you straighten your arms too soon it will make it much more challenging

*A straight arm inversion is considered advanced and requires core, grip and shoulder strength

*Invert with the fabric to the side of your body, not between your legs

1

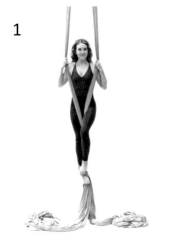

Begin from classic climb with your hands at shoulder height and elbows bent.

2

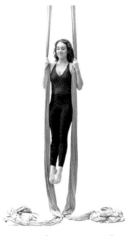

Release your feet bringing your legs and torso between the fabrics.

3

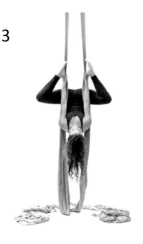

Invert brining your legs into a frog position.

4

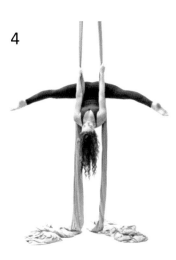

Extend your legs into a straddle. Retrace your path to exit. Repeat or rewrap in classic climb.

TIPS
*Passing your legs through a frog shape will make it easier to get your hips over your head. In time, work toward inverting with straight legs
*Do your best to keep your arms bent and elbows into your sides while inverting, if you straighten your arms too soon it will make it much more challenging
*A straight arm inversion is considered advanced and requires core, grip and shoulder strength
*Invert with the fabric on the outside of your hips, not between your legs

Single Thigh Wrap

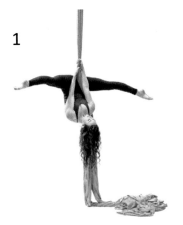

1

Begin from a straddle inversion with the tail on the right side.

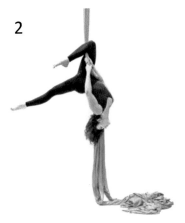

2

Hook your right knee above your hands, rotate your left leg behind you.

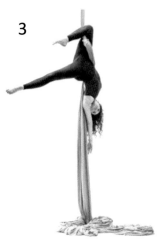

3

Release your left hand. With a back stroke motion reach behind you for the tail.

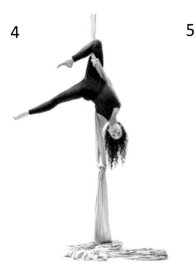

4

Grab the tail with your left hand, thumb pointing upward.

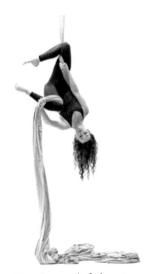

5

Bend your left knee toward your chest. Wrap your knee from the inside out.

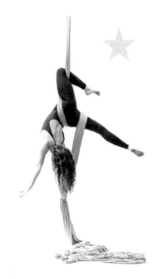

6

Hold the tail to prevent sliding.

7

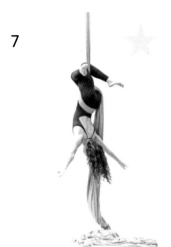

Option to cross your back leg over your hooked leg and release the tail.

8

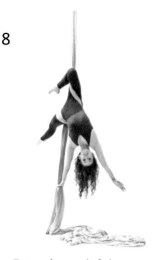

Extend your left leg behind you, holding the tail.

9

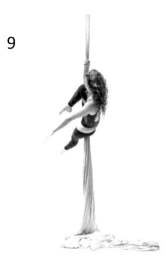

To exit, grip the fabric above your right knee with your right hand. Release the tail.

10

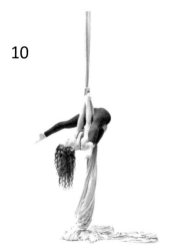

Place your left hand underneath your hooked knee. Release your right hand to unhook your right knee. Regrip with both hands and invert into a straddle.

11

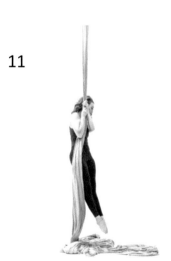

Pull up and lower your legs underneath you. Rewrap in classic climb or step down.

TIPS
*The single thigh wrap is a foundation skill for many more advanced aerial skills
*When learning this, don't climb up, invert off the floor for safety
*Make sure you don't hook your knee on top of your hands during step 2
*During step 5, keep your heel close to your tush and maintain a pointed foot to ensure an easy wrap
*Step 6 or 7 can both be the finished position
AKA: Catchers

FOOT LOCKS

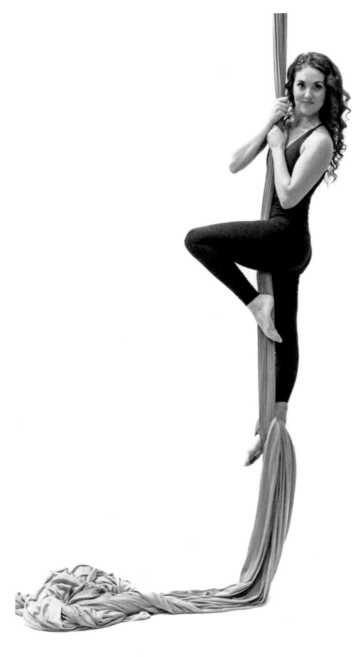

1

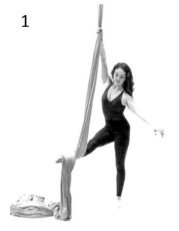

Wrap your leg around the fabric from the outside in and straighten your lifted leg.

2

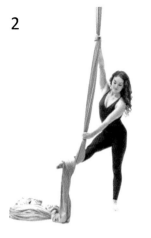

Grab the fabric next to your knee.

3

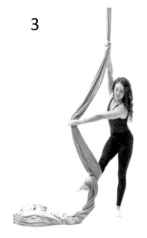

Pull the fabric to the side until it is in line with your hip.

4

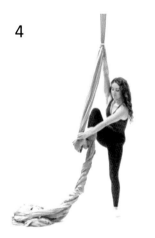

Reach the fabric across the top of your foot towards your pinky toe.

5

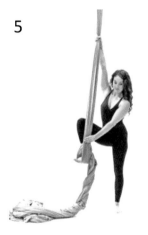

Step into the loop while placing the fabric on the arch of your foot.

TIPS
*It is common to wrap your foot incorrectly, make sure the pole end and tail of the fabric always end up on the inside of your arch
*The measurement of grabbing by your knee and pulling until the fabric is in line with your hip (step 3) will give you enough slack to comfortably step so the foot lock doesn't pinch
*If your foot is in pain you probably didn't give yourself enough slack to step in, or the fabric is twisted
*Repeat on your other side

AKA: Foot Knot

Single Foot Lock – Air Bound

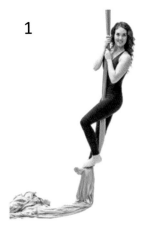

1

Begin from classic climb on the right side.

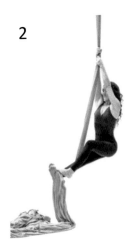

2

Reach your arms up and sit your hips back to form an L shape.

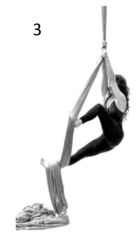

3

Lift your top left knee toward your chest. Internally rotate your leg and place the outside edge of your foot on the pole of the fabric.

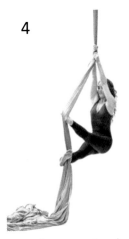

4

Lengthen your top leg and internally rotate your bottom leg. Aim the fabric over the top of your right foot using the outside edge of your left foot.

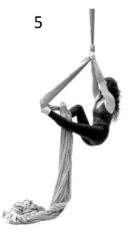

5

Continue to press the fabric across the top of your right foot as you bend your bottom right leg to step into the slack.

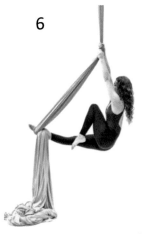

6

Release your left foot from the wrap.

7

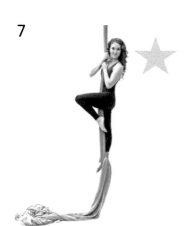

Pull up and stand on your foot lock.

8

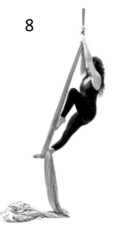

To exit, use the top of your left foot to push the foot lock off.

9

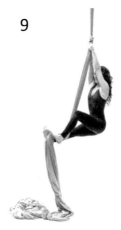

Let the foot lock fall off completely and re-wrap your feet in Classic Climb.

Alternate Way to Foot Lock

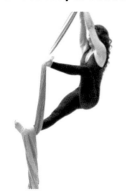

Externally rotate your top leg during steps 3-5.

TIPS

*When wrapping the single foot lock in the air, lift your top leg high to press the fabric across your foot so you have plenty of slack to step in

*Internally rotating your leg and using the outside of your foot to press the fabric (step 3-5) will be more accessible for most. As an alternate entry, it can be done externally rotating your leg and using the arch of your foot

*Repeat on your other side

AKA: Foot Knot

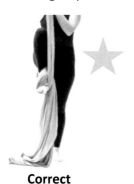

Correct

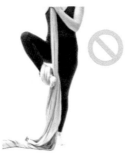

Incorrect

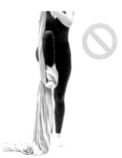

Incorrect

Single Foot Lock Positions

Side Tilt

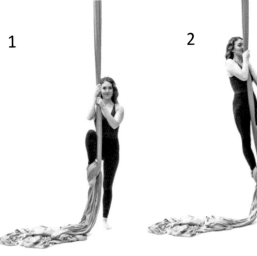

1

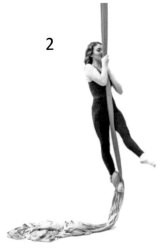

2

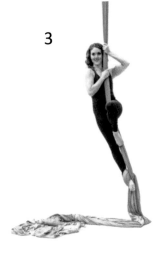

3

Begin from a single foot lock on your right.

Step up and or begin from a single foot lock in the air.

Place your left hand the height of the top of your head and your right in front of your chest on the pole of the fabric.

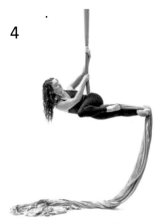

4

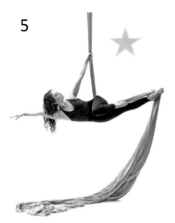

5

Begin leaning to the right placing your hip crease on the fabric and aiming your knee down.

Once you feel secure, reach your right arm out to the side.

TIPS
*To secure the position place the fabric in your hip crease and aim your knee downwards
*Placing your hand at the height of the top of your head ensures you arrive in a nice straight line when leaning to the side
*To exit, place both hands on the pole end and pull yourself back to an upright position
*Repeat on your other side

Back Arch Passé

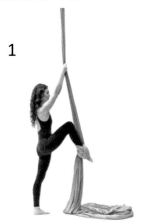

1

Begin from a single foot lock. Separate the fabrics.

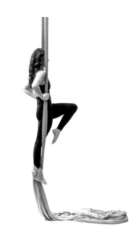

2

Step up. Place your hips between the fabrics. Move your hands one at time to waist level. Bend your knee toward your chest.

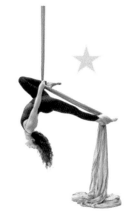

3

With a strong grip slowly arch back pressing your hips upward. Keep your knee toward your chest and opposite leg straight.

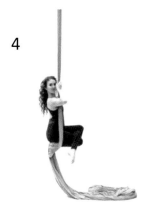

4

Bend your foot locked leg in between the fabrics and sit on your heel. Cross the opposite leg over.

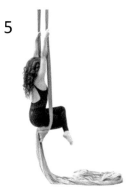

5

Reach your arms up high.

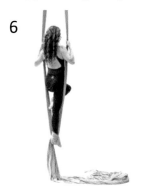

6

Use your arms and your supporting leg to stand up. To exit, step back and down.

TIPS

*The hand placement is important, make sure your hands are no lower than your waist or it may result in an accidental 360 flip backward!

*Make sure you have a strong grasp on the fabric and move slowly when arching back

*To come out in step 3, draw your chin to you chest as your bend your supporting leg to avoid feeling dizzy

AKA: Reverse Pendulum

Front Arch Passé

1

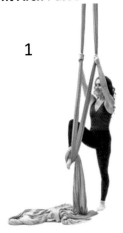

Begin from a single foot lock. Separate the fabrics.

2

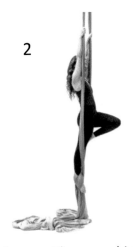

Step up. Place your hips between the fabrics. Reach your arms up high. Bend your knee toward your chest.

3

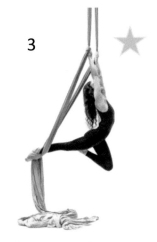

With a strong grip, pass your shoulders in front of the poles and begin to lean forward.

4

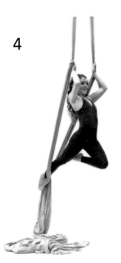

To come out, rotate your elbows forward and pull yourself back between the fabrics.

5

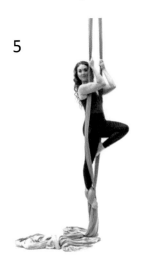

Move your elbows behind the poles of the fabric. To exit step back and down.

TIPS
*The transition from step 3-4 takes a lot of upper body strength to pull the shoulders back through
*Keep your foot locked leg pulled up and straight the entire time
*You can transition from this into Lay Back Arch

AKA: Forward Pendulum

Figure 8 Double Foot Locks – Floor Bound

1

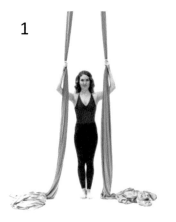

Begin in between
the fabrics.

2

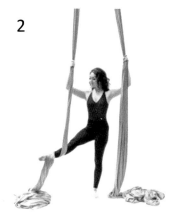

Wrap your right leg
outside around.

3

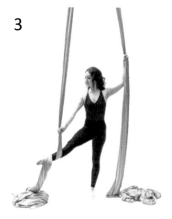

Grab the fabric by
your knee.

4

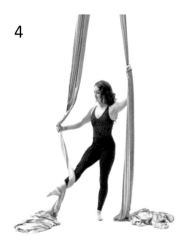

Pull the fabric until it is in
line with your hip to
create slack.

5

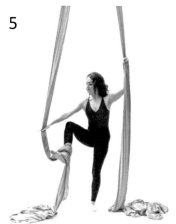

Reach the fabric across the
top of your foot and under
your arch.

6

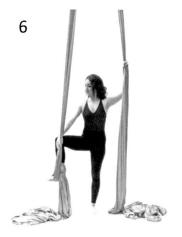

Step into the loop of
slack.

7

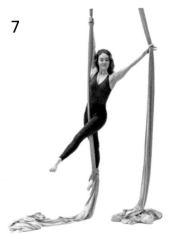

Step up on the right leg. Hold the opposite fabric in your left hand.

8

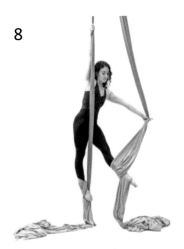

Grab the fabric by your knee, pull until it is in line with your hip to create slack.

9

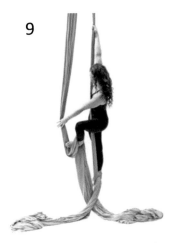

Reach the fabric across the top of your foot and under your arch. Begin bending your left knee.

10

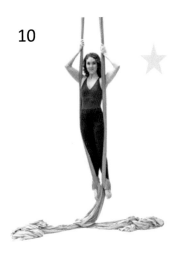

Step into the left loop of slack.

11

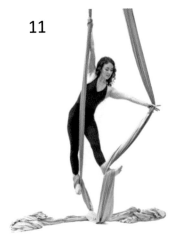

To exit, retrace your path. Take the left foot lock off by using your hand to unwrap it.

12

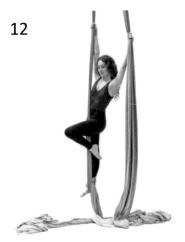

Hold the free fabric.

13

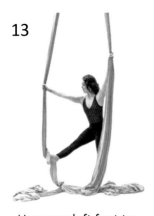

Use your left foot to pop your right foot lock off or simply unwrap by stepping down on the floor to take it off.

TIPS
*The second side can be tricky, be aware of how much fabric you are pulling that will help make your foot locks even
*Grab by your knee and pull the fabric approximately two feet so it is in line with your hip, that way you always have an even measurement when putting the second foot lock on
*Keep your body pressed against the fabric on the first side and your supporting arm reaching up high, you will feel more balanced
*No shaking or flailing to get the foot locks off. Instead, retrace your path by taking one off at a time and step down with control
*To exit figure 8 foot locks always step backward

Alternate Way to Put on the Second Foot Lock

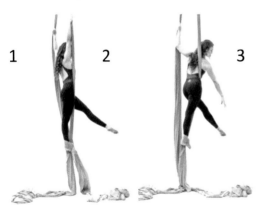

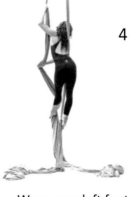

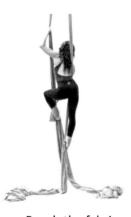

1

2

3

4

Start from Step 7 on pg. 46. Step up on the right leg. Hold the opposite fabric in your left hand.

Pass your right arm in front of the pole, place the pole of the fabric behind your right armpit.

Wrap your left foot outside around the free fabric. Grab the free fabric with your right hand next to your knee. Pull until it is line with your hip.

Reach the fabric across the top of your foot and under your arch. Bend your left knee and step into the loop.

Figure 8 Double Foot Locks – Air Bound

1

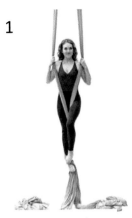

Begin from the classic climb with the fabrics apart.

2

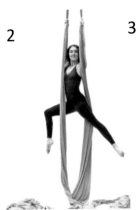

Transfer your weight into your arms and take your feet off the fabric.

3

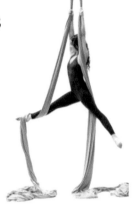

Wrap your right leg from the outside around.

4

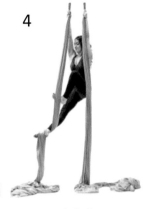

Use your left foot to press the fabric across the top of your right foot.

5

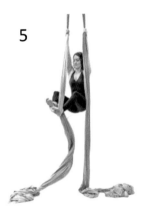

Bend your right leg to step into the foot lock.

6

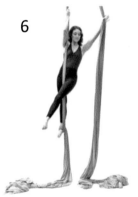

Wrap your left leg outside around. Grab the fabric by your knee pull to the side.

7

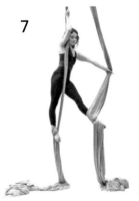

Reach the fabric across the top of your foot and under your arch.

8

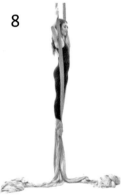

Step into the left loop of slack.

Exit Option #1 Flex Your Feet

1
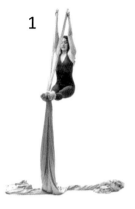
Straighten your arms and drop your hips back.

2
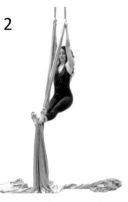
Flex your feet firmly to allow the wraps to come off your feet.

3
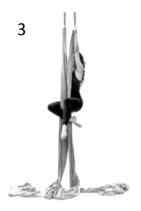
Begin rewrapping your feet.

4
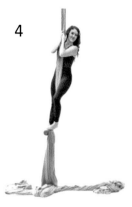
Step on the fabric in a climbing position.

Exit Option #2 – Pull Up

1
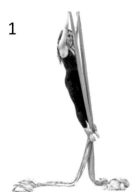
Reach your arms up high.

2
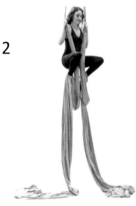
Bend your knees bringing your heels toward your tush.

3
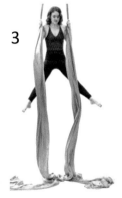
Extend your legs back and down.

4
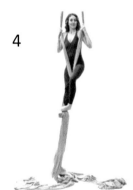
Wrap your feet in a climbing position.

TIPS
*The air bound foot locks can be done from bent arms or straight arms
*During step 2 pass your torso between the fabrics and watch that the fabrics don't get tangled together when putting the first foot lock on
*Steps 6-8 are the same as the floor bound version

AKA: Double Foot Knots

Egg Beater Double Foot Locks

1

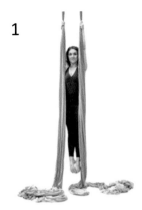

Hang with straight arms between the fabrics.

2

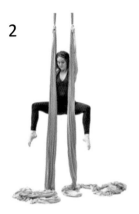

Begin to open your legs placing the tails in the front of your upper thighs.

3

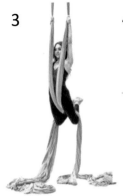

Pass your feet between the fabrics bringing your heels close to your tush.

4

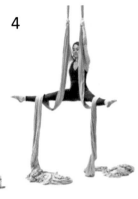

Circle your lower legs open into a straddle

5

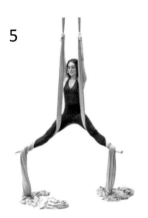

Repeat steps 2-3 to complete two wraps.

6

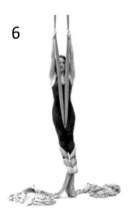

Draw your legs and feet together.

7

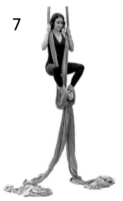

Pull up, bend your knees with your feet pressing together to create loops of slack under your feet.

8

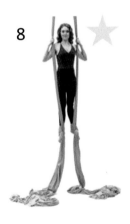

Step back and down into the loops.

Exit Option #1 Step Forward One Foot Lock at a Time

1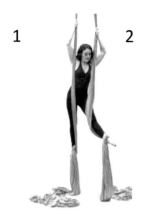

Begin stepping forward to release one foot lock.

2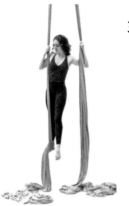

Hold the free fabric.

3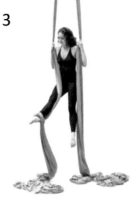

Step forward to release the second foot lock.

4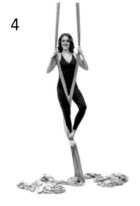

Step on the fabric in a climbing position.

Exit Option #2 – Closed Fabric

1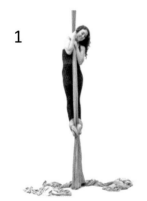

Hold the fabrics together with the poles on the inside of your knees.

2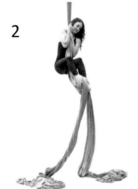

Lift your knees up, forward and down to release the foot locks.

3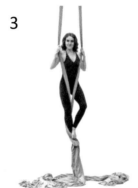

Wrap your feet in a climbing position.

Floor Bound Drill for Precise Wraps

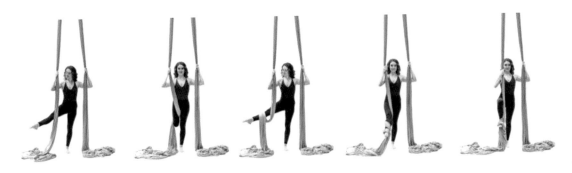

Alternate Entry from Bent Arms

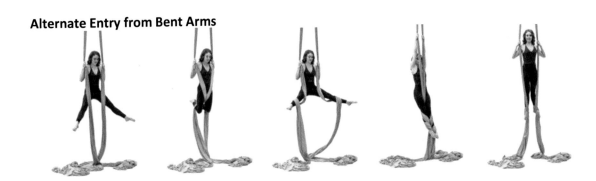

TIPS
*On step 3 (page 50), emphasize bringing your heels toward your tush as much as you can, this will place the fabric high on the back of your knees where you need it
*The pathway of the legs is back, side, back and feet together
*Practice wrapping one leg at a time off of the floor to understand the pathway of the wrap before you exhaust your arms trying it in the air
*To take the foot locks off, place the fabric on the inside of your legs, bend your knees while stepping forward and down in a prancing motion

AKA: Dance Wrap

Foot Lock Splits

Front Splits

1
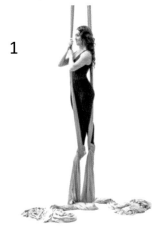

Begin from either version of double foot locks. Turn to face one fabric. Place your hands on the front fabric.

2
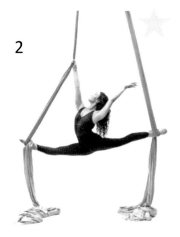

Lower into a split with square hips and fully lengthened legs. Option to release your bottom hand and extend your arm to frame your face.

3
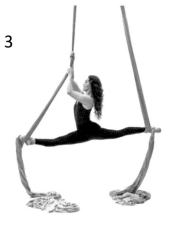

Place both hands on the front fabric and begin pulling up out of your split.

4
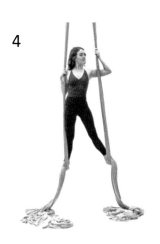

Stand up and begin to transition to the other fabric moving one hand at a time.

5
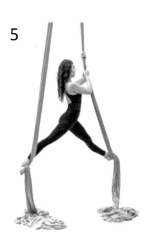

Place your hands on the front fabric and begin lowering into a split on your opposite side.

6
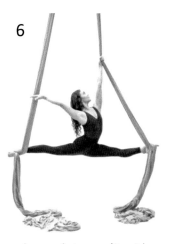

Lower into a split with square hips and fully lengthened legs.

Incorrect Back Leg

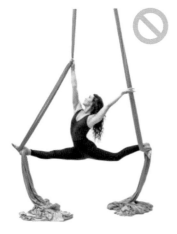

TIPS
*You do not need to be able to do full splits to do this, aerial splits will help your splits tremendously as long as your leg muscles are active
*Keep your hips squared off to the front for a more effective stretch
*Make sure you have thoroughly warmed up your splits prior to doing air bound splits
*Be careful on the transition to the 2nd side on your front splits, it's easy to lose balance
*Keep your feet pointed throughout

Cross Back Straddle Inversion

1
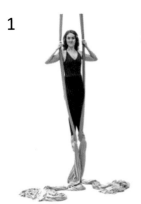

2
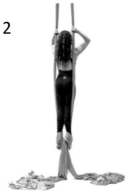

3
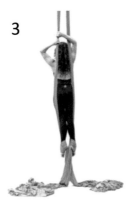

4
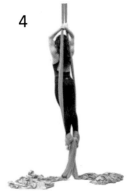

Begin from double foot locks.

Bring your left arm in front of the fabric. Reach your right arm forwards.

Circle your right arm behind the right fabric to grab the left.

Switch your left hand to the front of the right fabric forming an X behind you.

5

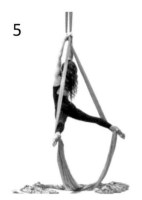

Arch forward, open your legs behind you.

6

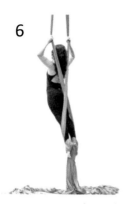

Pull your arms to the side while closing your legs.

7

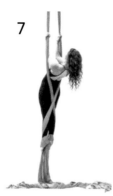

Pass your head and shoulders between the fabrics.

8

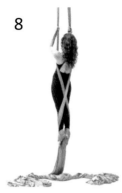

Place your arms on the opposite side of the fabric one at a time.

9

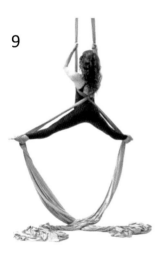

Turn out your legs and begin to straddle until you feel the X move above your tush.

10

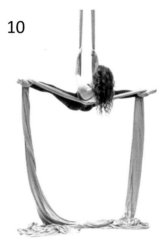

Pull up, tuck your pelvis under and push the fabric forward while lifting your legs wide to the side.

11

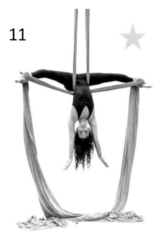

Arrive in an inverted straddle. Press your inner thighs against the poles of fabric and release your hands.

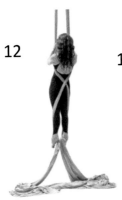

12

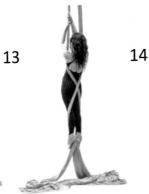

13

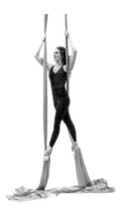

14

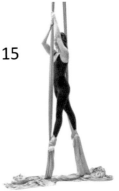

15

To come out grab the poles and bring your shoulders up. Keep your legs straight, close them underneath you.

Reach across with one arm and grab the opposite fabric.

Place both hands on the left fabric. Bring your shoulders out of the X.

Reach across with your other arm.

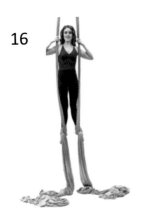

16

Face in between the fabrics with one hand on each fabric.

TIPS
*Even foot locks are key to the success of this skill
*Practice steps 1-8 on the floor without foot locks on so you understand the pathway of your hand placement prior to doing it in the air
*In the transition from step 6 to 7, make sure your legs are together. Open legs will make it difficult to get your head and shoulders through the X
*The transition from steps 9 to 11 can be challenging. Be mindful that your legs are turning out from your hips, your lower abs are engaged and slightly tuck your pelvis under to initiate the inversion
*If you have very open hips you may not need to pull up during step 10, you can simply push the fabric forward to invert
*There are many ways to get the X on your back, this is one of more straight forward entries
*To exit, always grab the fabric that is closest to your back

AKA: Straddle X Back, Butterfly

The Scorpion

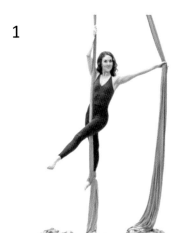

1

Place a single foot lock on your right foot. Hold the left free fabric.

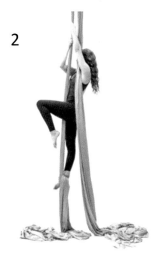

2

Place the free fabric in front of your left armpit and grab with your left hand.

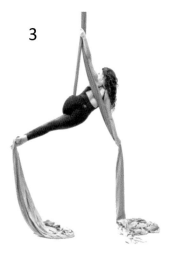

3

Lean to the right reaching behind you for the free fabric with your right hand.

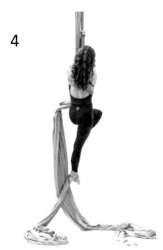

4

Using your right arm circle the tail around your waist until it is on the outside of your left hip.

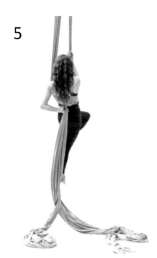

5

Switch your hands so your right hand holds the pole end, your left hand holds the tail. Press your left hand holding the tail into your lower back.

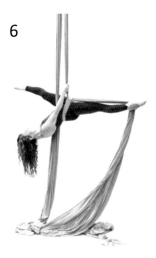

6

Lean back and extend your left leg as you continue to press the tail into your lower back.

7

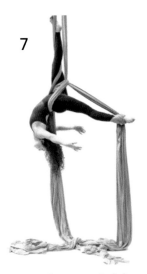

Crochet your left leg outside around the left fabric. Sickle your left foot around the pole to secure the position. Once secured release your hands.

8

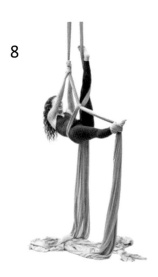

Climb up the right fabric, keep your left foot sickling and pressing into the pole.

9

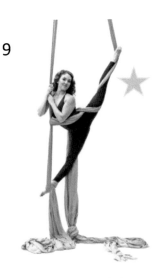

Rotate your left leg behind you arriving in and *arabesque* or *attitude* position.

10

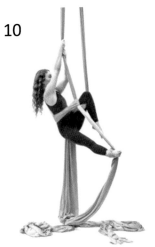

Keep your hands in the same place. Drop your hips back and bend your left knee.

11

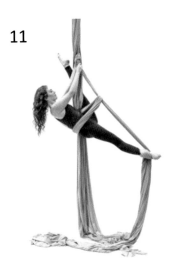

Extend your left leg to release the wrap.

12

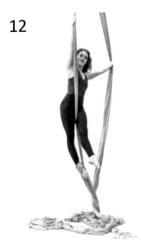

Stand up and allow the wrap to fall off from around your waist.

Alternate Final Pose– Less Flexibility Required

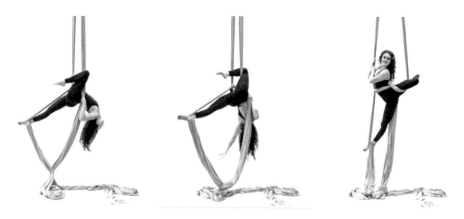

TIPS
*Stretch your back and hip flexors well before doing this
*Always begin with the tail of the fabric on the opposite side of the foot that is locked
*Your top foot needs to stay sickled and pressing into the pole as you rotate into the final attitude or arabesque position in step 8. Normally sickled feet are incorrect, since we are using it as a leverage point it is an exception to the rule
*Try this low to the floor in case you need to step down before taking it higher

 AKA: Rebecca Split

"You are never too old to set another goal
or to dream a new dream."
C.S. Lewis

AERIAL PROGRESSIONS

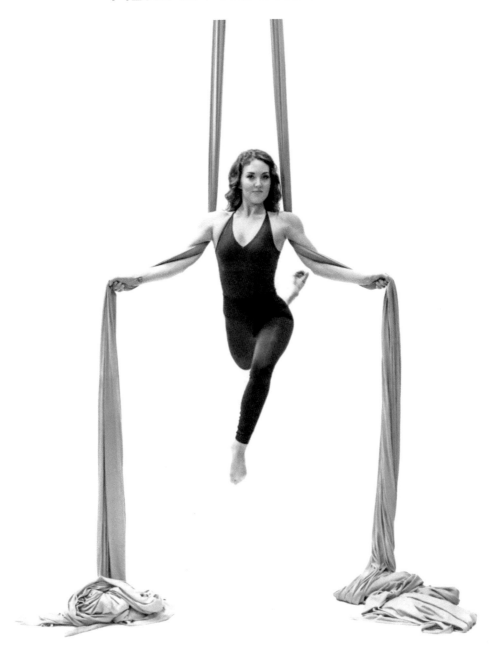

Hip Key

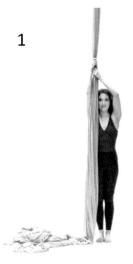

1

Begin with the fabric on your right side.

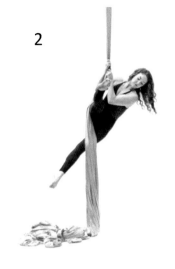

2

Pull up with your arms and scissor your legs with your right leg forward and left leg back. Catch the fabric between your upper thighs.

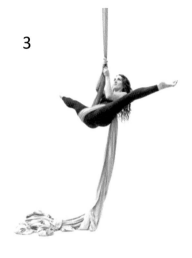

3

Pass through a straddle keeping your arms bent to support you.

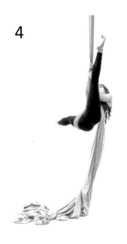

4

Aim your left leg upward toward to pole of the fabric to ensure the fabric falls above your top hip.

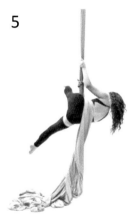

5

Continue the pathway of your left leg, begin pressing your top hip into the pole of the fabric.

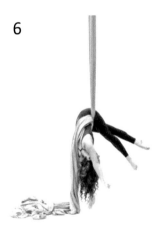

6

Arrive in a scissor position with your legs, top hip pressing into the pole and your head lower than your tush.

Alternate Entry– Less Flexibility Required – Knee to Chest

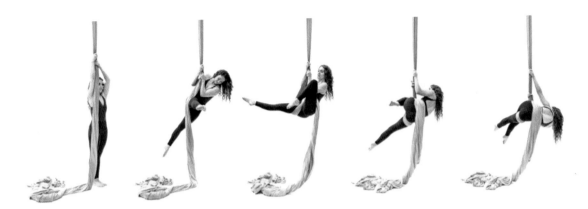

Incorrect Hip Key Position   **Correct Hip Key Position**

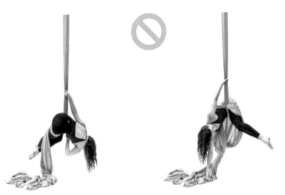   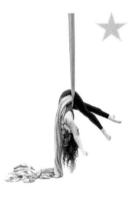

TIPS
*When beginning, this may end up looking like a knee key or thigh key, both are incorrect. To avoid the fabric ending up too low you must lift your outside leg up high enough so the fabric falls above your hip
*Do your best to maintain bent arms with your elbows into your sides when passing through the scissor and straddle, if your arms straighten too soon you will lose height
*Once you've tried it from the floor, try it in the air from a climbing position
*The hip key is an important foundational skill for more advanced tricks
*"Scissor, straddle, scissor" is a fun mantra to use when learning this
*This skill can be a brain teaser! You are not alone ☺
AKA: Hip Lock

Double Ankle Hang

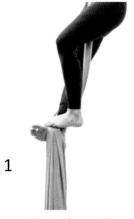

1

Begin from the classic climb on your right.

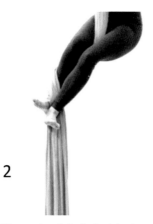

2

Place the fabric behind your left heel. Circle your feet to the right with your feet side by side.

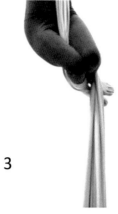

3

Continue to circle right until the fabric is around your ankles once and the tail is on the outside of your right foot.

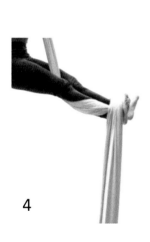

4

Begin to pike your hips back and walk your hands down aiming the pole of the fabric between your feet.

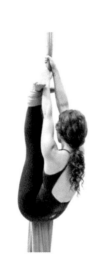

5

Firmly flex your feet arriving in a pike position.

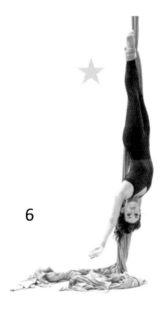

6

Release your hands and hang upside down. Once you are secured in position, point your feet.

7

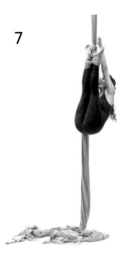

To exit, sit up and reach for the pole above your feet or climb up the tail. If you began from a right side climb, keep the tail to the right.

8

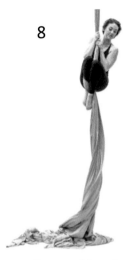

Pull up and bend your knees forward and down.

9

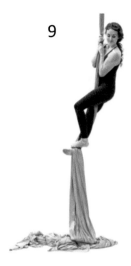

Wrap your feet in a climbing position.

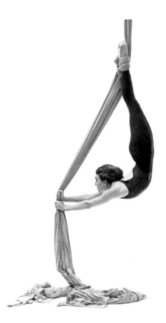

TIPS
 *Practice steps 1-5 low to the floor to make sure you understand the wrap before trying it up higher
*The feet must stay side by side the entire time with no space between them
*If you began from a right side climb, the tail must be to the right side to exit smoothly
*You can use the double ankle to perform sit ups for conditioning
*There are a variety of shapes you can make in the ankle hang in addition to spinning!

AKA: Coffin Hang

1

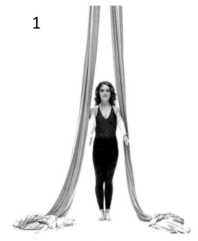

Begin standing between the fabrics with your arms reaching forward.

2

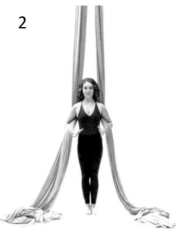

Begin to circle your arms outside around.

3

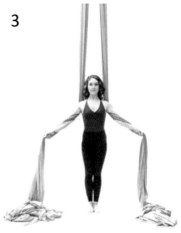

Wrap once, lengthen your arms and grab the fabrics.

4

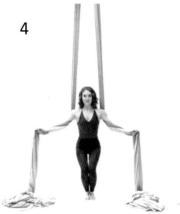

Bend your knees and begin to transfer your weight into your arms. Draw your shoulder blades down your back.

5

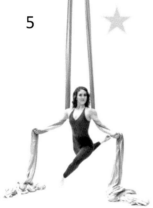

Lift your feet off the floor and arrange your legs in a stag position or place your knees together side by side. To exit, simply step down.

TIPS
*When you shift your weight into your arms, most likely your shoulders will want to hunch forward, think about using your back muscles to support you versus your neck and wrists
*There are many leg variations, this is just one!
*Keep practicing this on the floor version before taking it in the air
*This can feel uncomfortable on the back of the armpits. If your skin is tender, wear a long sleeve shirt

AKA: Iron T

Iron Cross in the Air

1

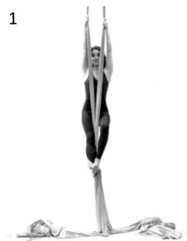

Begin from classic climb with split fabrics.

2

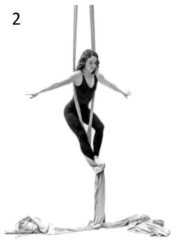

Pass your shoulders between the poles one arm at a time.

3

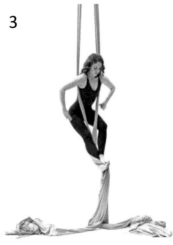

Drop your hips back and begin to bend your arms.

4

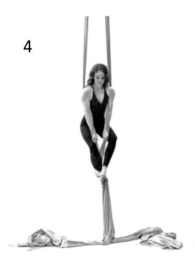

Pass your hands in the space between your upper thighs and the fabric. Circle your wrists around the fabrics.

5

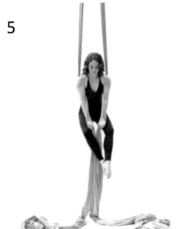

Maintain a strong grip. Release your feet and begin to open your arms to the side.

6

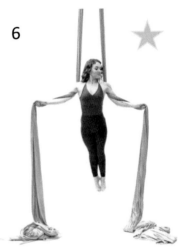

Open your arms to the side as wide as you can control forming a T shape.

7	8	9

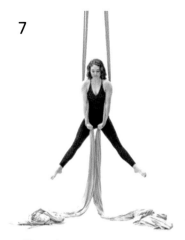 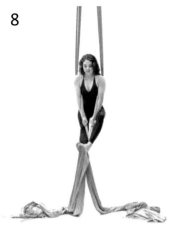 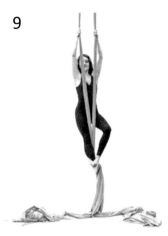

To exit, press your arms forward and down.	Lift your knees up high and wrap your feet in classic climb.	Reach one arm up at a time and pass your shoulders behind the pole ends.

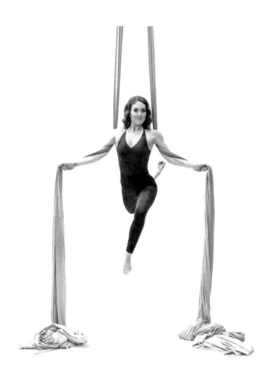

TIPS

*Move your arms open from your upper back not from your wrists

*In the beginning your arms may not make it to the full iron cross position, that is ok

*Be careful when trying this in the air for the first time, it is demanding on the upper body and wrists

*There are many leg variations you can do in the iron cross as well as movements such as walking in the air

*When exiting lift your knees up high before re-wrapping your feet in step 8 to avoid an armpit burn

*This position makes you look very strong! ☺

AKA: Iron T

CONDITIONING

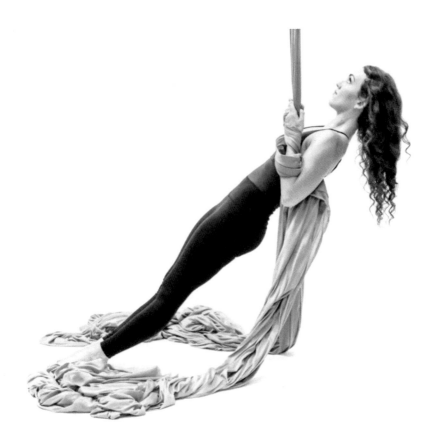

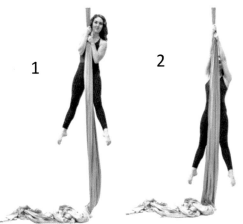

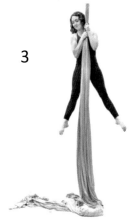

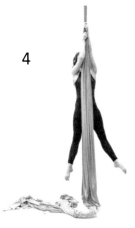

1 Begin from a climbing position with your right hand on top. Release your feet and draw your elbows into your sides. Hold for 10-30 seconds.

2 Slowly elongate your arms until your top arm is straight. Hold for 10-30 seconds.

3 Begin from a climbing position with your left hand on top. Release your feet and draw your elbows into your sides. Hold for 10-30 seconds.

4 Slowly elongate your arms until your top arm is straight. Hold for 10-30 seconds.

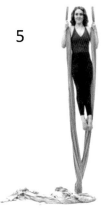

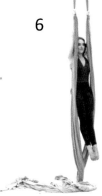

5 Begin from a climbing position with split fabrics. Release your feet and draw your elbows into your hands. Hold for 10-30 seconds.

6 Slowly elongate your arms until your top arm is straight. Hold for 10-30 seconds.

TIPS
*The starting position in steps 1, 3 & 5 draw your elbows into your hips, keep your color bones wide and neck long
*When lowering to straight arms move slowly with control working the negative pull up action
*This exercise will improve your upper body endurance and strength
*Maintain hollow body throughout all positions

AKA: Six Hangs

Hammock Knot Conditioning

Supported Tuck Lifts

1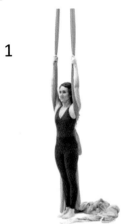

2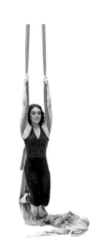

3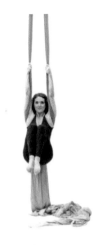

Begin tying a hammock knot. Place it behind you like you would a backpack for support.

Transfer your weight into your hands and lift your feet up. Bend your knees.

Draw your knees into your chest. Hold for 5-10 seconds. Slowly lower with control. Repeat 5-10x.

Supported Straddle Inversions

1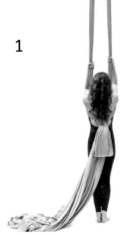

2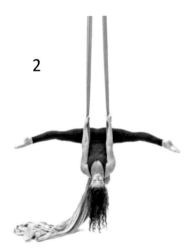

3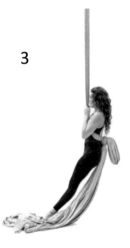

Begin with the hammock knot behind you for support.

Invert into a straddle passing through a frog position or keep your legs straight.

Lift your chest up and lower your legs underneath you without touching the floor. Repeat 5-10x.

Supported Pike Lifts

1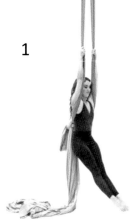

2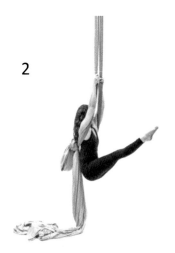

3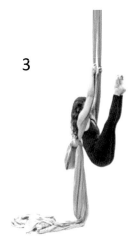

Begin with the hammock knot behind you for support. Transfer your weight into your hands and lift your legs slightly in front of you.

Tuck your hips under to initiate lifting your legs up to the front.

Continue to lift as high as you can keeping your legs tight and straight. Lower to step 1 with control. Repeat 5-10x.

TIPS
*The hammock knot supports some of your weight so you can perform the conditioning skills with assistance and focus on correct technique, alignment and perform more reps than you could without it
*For each exercise, focus on using your core strength to lift your legs up versus using momentum
*Inhale to begin each rep, exhale at the challenging part of the exercise. For example, for supported tuck and pike lifts, inhale to begin, exhale as you lift your legs up
*When beginning, 5-10 reps is plenty for most. As you gain more strength add more reps or multiple sets of 5-10

Supported Arm Climb

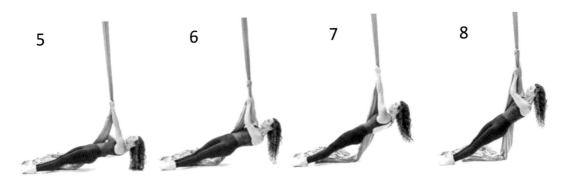

1 Begin standing holding the fabric with your hands approx. in line with the top of your head.

2 **3** **4** Keep your feet in the same place, lean back until your arms are straight. Draw your abs in and squeeze your legs and glutes together for stability. Begin walking down the fabric hand over hand.

5 **6** **7** **8** Continue to walk down until you are approximately one foot from the floor. Walk your hands back up until you are back at step 2. Repeat.

TIPS
*Maintain hollow body position throughout for stability
*Try to keep your lower body still as you climb up and down
*This is a great preparation exercise for eventual no leg climbs
*Start with 2-3 reps and add more as your strength increases

Lat Pulls

1

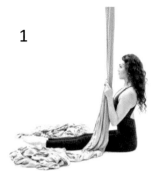

Begin seated with your legs straight out in front of you.

2

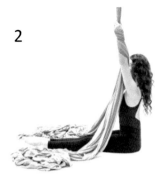

Circle your arms upward around the fabric from the outside in. Once or twice for more support.

3

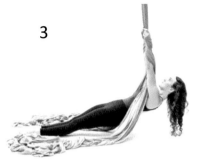

Lean your shoulders back and lift your hips up.

4

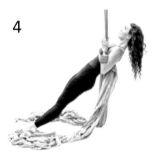

Begin drawing your shoulders down and back as you bend your elbows past your ribcage.

5

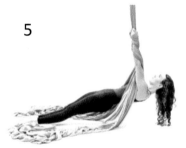

Lower to the starting position with control. Repeat 10x.

TIPS
*Maintain hollow body position throughout for stability
*If you are working with stretchy fabric you may need to reach your arms up ever higher before pulling to accommodate the stretch
*When bending your elbows keep your ribcage drawing together in the front
*Inhale to begin, exhale to pull
*If this is too challenging, it can be done from standing

AT HOME CONDITONING

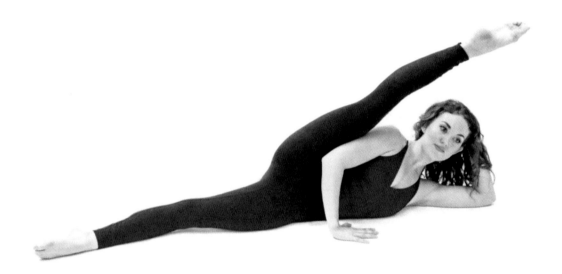

AT HOME GUIDE In order to progress more rapidly is it important to keep up with your strength and flexibility training on the days when you aren't at aerial class. In the at home guide, you will learn simple yet effective movements that will help you excel in your aerial classes. Keep in mind it's not the quantity but the quality. Begin with doing as many as you can with proper form and work your way up to doing at least 10 of each. In the hand weight section use 3 to 5 pound weights.

Leg Lifts

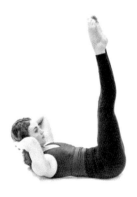

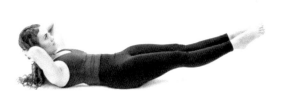

Begin laying on your back with your hands behind your head, shoulders off the floor and legs pointing upward. Legs slightly turned out and squeezing together.

Keep your abdominals pulling in and up as you lower your legs as far as you can without arching your back off the floor. Repeat.
Targets: Abdominals

Supine Ab Straddle

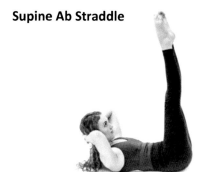

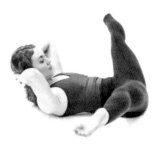

Begin laying on your back with your hands behind your head, shoulders off the floor and legs pointing upward. Legs slightly turned out and squeezing together.

Keep your legs turned out from your hips as you open your legs outward into a straddle. Repeat.
Targets: Abdominals, stretches & strengthens inner thighs

Side Laying Battements:

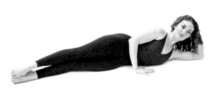

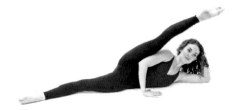

Lay on your side with your legs together, turned out and slightly in front of you.

Keep your legs straight and turned out from your hips as you lift your top leg up. Lower back down. Repeat.
Targets: Hips, outer thigh & stretches inner thighs

Push Ups

Triceps Push Ups

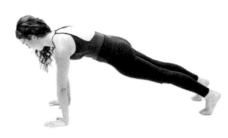

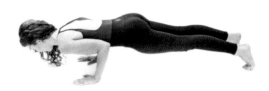

Begin from a plank position with your hands underneath your shoulders.

Maintain the same position in your torso as you lower down into a push up with your elbows into your sides. Be sure not to go past 90 degrees.
Targets: Triceps

Tricep Extensions

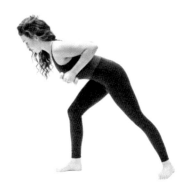 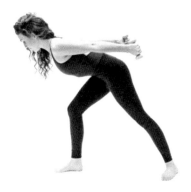

Stand in a staggered lunge position.
Elongate your spine and hug your
elbows into your sides.

Extend your arms back. Repeat.
Targets: Triceps

Lat Pull Downs

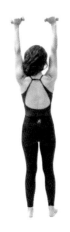 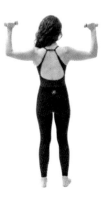

Begin with your arms open to the
side with elbows lifted in line with
your shoulders.

Extend your arms upward. Repeat.
Targets: Latissimus Dorsi

Rotator Cuff

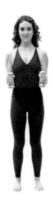 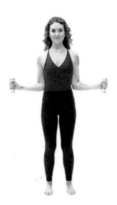

Begin with your elbows into your sides and forearms at a 90 degree angle.

Press your elbows into your sides as you open your arms outward. Repeat.
Targets: Shoulder & Chest Muscles

Grip Strengthener

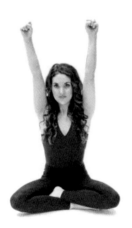 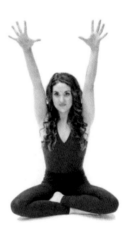

Reach your arms up and open your hands wide.

Close your hands tightly into a fist. Continue to quickly open and close your hands. Repeat for 60-90 seconds.
Targets: Grip Strength & Forearms

Pull Ups & Chin Ups

The number one exercise to improve your strength for aerial is pull ups and chin ups. Below are exercises you can do at home with a pull up bar in your doorway, at the gym, on monkey bars or using a lyra or trapeze. Any type of pull up movement is a difficult task. If you need an extra boost put a pull up band around the bar or place a chair underneath you to step up on.

Consistency is key when working toward achieving pull ups! Begin with a few assisted pull ups. When you feel your strength increase, try it without the band. Spending just 10 minutes a day on the exercises to follow, will make a huge difference in your strength. Please use extreme caution when using doorway pull up bars. Make sure it is fully secure before hanging on it.

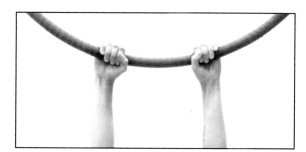

Pull Up Grip: Overhand grip with your palms facing away. The more difficult of the two grips.

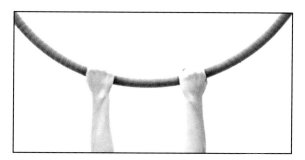

Chin Up Grip: Underhand grip with your palms facing toward you. This grip tends to be easier for most due to the biceps being more involved.

Shoulder Shrugs

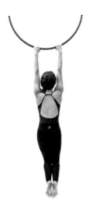

Hang from the bar with straight arms using a pull up grip. Engage your abdominals to lengthen your lower back. Pull your shoulders away from your ears.

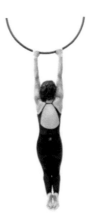

Shrug your shoulders up towards your ears keeping your arms straight. Pull your shoulders back down. Repeat.
Targets: Trapezius & surrounding shoulder muscles

Hollow Body Hang

Tuck Holds

Pike Holds

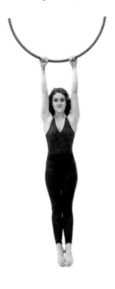

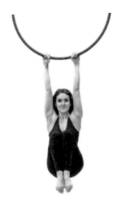

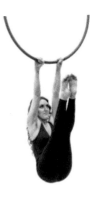

Hang from the bar with straight arms. Engage your abdominals to lengthen your lower back. Squeeze your legs together and point your feet. Hold.

Begin from the straight arm hang. Tuck your knees toward your chest. Hold for 5-10 seconds, straighten your legs back to your starting position.

Begin from the straight arm hang. Press your legs together and lift them in front of you into a pike. Hold for a few seconds, lower your legs to your staring position.
Targets: Abs, Latissimus Dorsi

Negative Chin Ups & Pull Ups

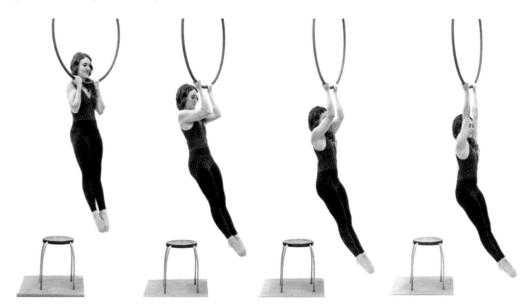

Place a sturdy chair to the side of the pull up bar, trapeze or lyra. Step up on the chair, pull your chin above the bar and lower down over the course of 10 seconds. Step back on the chair and repeat. This can be done in both the chin up and pull up grips. The chair raises the floor so there is less distance for you to pull up.

Incorrect Position   **Correct Position**

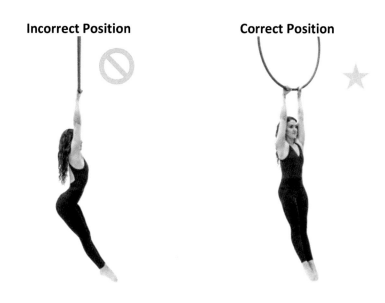

Pull Ups

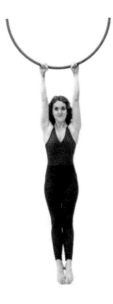

Hang from the bar with straight arms using the pull up grip. Engage your abdominals to lengthen your lower back. Begin to pull your shoulders down your back to initiate the pull up action.

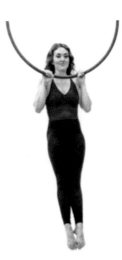

Continue to pull until your chin is above the bar. Lower down with control. Repeat.
Targets: Latissimus Dorsi & Triceps

Chin Ups

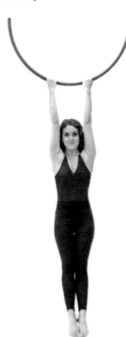

Hang from the bar with straight arms using the chin up grip. Engage your abdominals to lengthen your lower back. Begin to pull your shoulders down your back and bend your elbows into your sides.

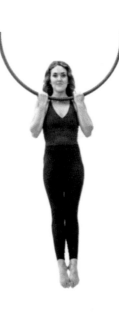

Keep pulling until your chin is above the bar. Lower down with control. Repeat.
Targets: Latissimus Dorsi & Biceps

ACKNOWLEGMENTS

The author, Jill Franklin, would like to thank the following for their assistance with the production of this book:

TC Franklin – Photographer
www.tcfranklin.com

A very special thank you to all of the teachers of movement throughout my life, I have learned something unique from each and everyone one of you.
You have helped become who I am today.

Many thanks to my aerial students and followers who inspired me to write this book.
This is for you!

ABOUT THE AUTHOR

Jill Franklin is the founder of Aerial Physique. She is also a celebrity trainer and author of numerous books including *Beginners Guide to Aerial Silk, Intermediate Guide to Aerial Silk, Aerial Physique FIT, Aerial Silks Coloring Book & Cirque Coloring Book*. She maintains a highly sought after You Tube channel and a web based video site, Aerial Physique TV. Jill is also a clothing designer with a line featuring the J-Boss & K-Boss Jumpsuits, specifically designed for aerial work! Jill has a certifiable Aerial Teacher Training Program based in the U.S. On a global scale, Jill renews her vigorously intense teacher training course to hundreds of eager students throughout Europe, Thailand and China. Jill maintains complete course offerings annually in countries such as Austria, Italy, Germany, Switzerland, Thailand and others. Jill's Aerial Physique Inc., has a new World Headquarters in Shenyang, China. It is the largest aerial teacher training venue of its kind, helping develop hundreds of aerial instructors from across the globe. Jill's definitive and precise teaching expertise, enables instructors to better teach their own students with new, innovative and exciting aerial silks skills with its ever-changing artistic format.

Jill has an extensive background in ballet along with certifications in Pilates and yoga all which encompass her Aerial Physique technique. She has a 5-Star rated studio based in Los Angeles. Since its inception in 2012, her studio continually attracts thousands of aspiring aerialists from around the world. Jill's expertise spans through ten years of aerial experience and she's been a featured aerialist for dozens of events and productions throughout the world. Her performances include celebrity filled galas and events throughout Los Angeles and surrounding cities. Jill has gracefully mesmerized audiences with her stunning performances in productions seen on the cruise ship Royal Caribbean's Oasis of the Seas as a featured nightly act. She has been seen in aerial productions at The Arlington Theatre-Santa Barbara, Waikiki Shell-Honolulu, Balboa Theatre-San Diego and many others.

Aerial Physique has been televised on the TODAY Show and Jill has been featured in People Magazine, Muscle and Fitness Hers, Vogue, Shape and Latina Magazine. Additional articles and media coverage featuring Jill's work can be found in Prevention Magazine, Good Day LA, Inside Edition, Yahoo Celebrity, ABC 7 LA and many other media outlets. Jill is always excited to share her knowledge and expertise with you and help you live a life full of Beauty, Grace and Strength.

Jill began the Aerial Physique Teacher Training program in 2014 after noticing a need for well-trained instructors in her own studio. Since then, her program has expanded internationally gaining wide-spread acclaim with an enormous following of aspiring aerial instructors.

The Aerial Physique Book Collection

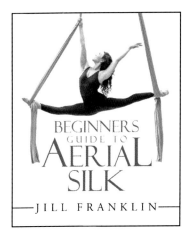

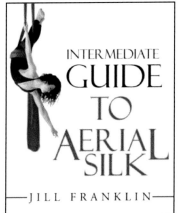

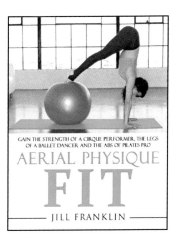

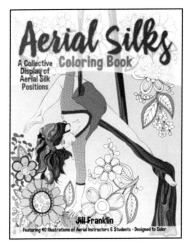

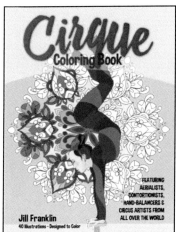

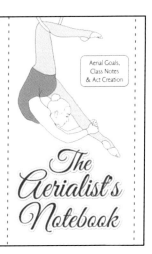

Available on www.amazon.com & www.aerialphysique.com

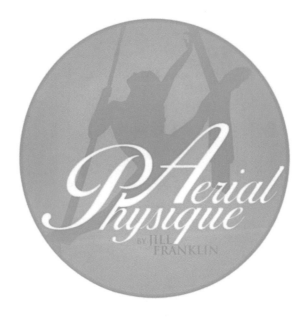

Aerial Physique offers teacher training programs and workshops worldwide.

www.aerialphysique.com

Contact Aerial Physique:
info@aerialphysique.com
1-800-208-2246

Made in the USA
Middletown, DE
03 June 2023

32011035R00055